PRAISE FOR

SHE WANTS A RING—AND I DON'T WANNA CHANGE A THING

"I loved this book! It is what every woman should understand about
her potential husband so she can help him over the obstacles of getting married. Barron gives simple, realistic solutions to what previously seemed like insurmountable hurdles."

—Nita Tucker, author of *How Not to Stay Single*

"What a relief to read a wise book that is also witty, daring, and playful.
James Barron has lived the problem—and solved it—not just
for himself but for a lot of guys. Barron travels the male psyche—
heretofore the rockiest of roads—and makes the journey fun and
easy."
—Pepper Schwartz, Ph.D., author
of *Everything You Know About Love
and Sex Is Wrong* and *American Couples*

She Wants a Ring 💍

—and I Don't Wanna Change a Thing

Also by
James Douglas Barron

*She's Having a Baby—and
I'm Having a Breakdown*

*She's Had a Baby—and
I'm Having a Meltdown*

She Wants a Ring🔔

Ring💍

—and I Don't Wanna Change a Thing

*How a Man Can Overcome His Fears
of Commitment and Marriage*

James Douglas Barron

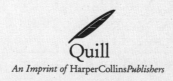

Quill
An Imprint of HarperCollinsPublishers

HarperCollins books may be purchased for educational, business, or sales promotional use. For information please write: Special Markets Department, HarperCollins Publishers Inc., 10 East 53rd Street, New York, NY 10022.

Designed by The Book Design Group / Matt Perry Ratto

Library of Congress Cataloging-in-Publication Data

Barron, James Douglas.
   She wants a ring—and I don't wanna change a thing: how a man can overcome his fears of commitment and marriage / James Douglas Barron.—1st ed.
        p. cm.
   ISBN 0-688-17950-9 (alk. paper)
   1. Man-woman relationships. 2. Commitment (Psychology). 3. Men—Psychology. I. Title: How a man can overcome his fears of commitment and marriage. II. Title.
HQ801 .B33 2001
306.7—dc21   00-059447

---

01 02 03 04 05 ❖ / RRD 10 9 8 7 6 5 4 3 2 1

For Jeannette, Isabelle, and Benjamin

Contents

Introduction

I ALWAYS IMAGINED IT WOULD BE EASY. I would take one glance at a woman and know she was The One. We'd go on hot dates that would lead to sizzling nights. I'd totally lose interest in other women (no twitch of a skirt or bob of a breast would capture my gaze). I would be whacked out in love, floating upside down and sideways . . . until one day, months later, under twinkling stars, I'd murmur, "Will you marry me?" She'd throw her arms around me and yelp, "Yes, yes, yes, yes, *yes!*" We'd tell our parents, and they'd be elated. Then, completely composed, we'd plan a small wedding under a big tree, where we'd dance and frolic, and well-behaved friends and relatives would nod and whisper, "Perfect."

Well, it wasn't quite like that.

Amazingly, the first part of my fairy-tale vision came true. I met my bride-to-be in a New York City elevator not far from one of the busiest intersections in the world, Fifty-Seventh Street and Fifth

Avenue. With my heart pounding, I said hello, and she smiled back. We flirted shamelessly for an hour, I was exalted and got back to work late, we started dating, fell wildly in love, and within a few weeks were talking about what color eyes our babies would have.

There was just one minor detail: Like millions of men before me, I couldn't get over the Is She The One? Problem, the Forever? Problem, the No Other Women for the Rest of My Life? Problem, the How Do We Know We'll Love Each Other When We're Shriveled Up Old Raisins? Problem. She could see the future; I couldn't.

Suddenly, everyone said I had a "commitment problem." I heard lots of advice. From her mother: "If you're not serious, let her go." From my best friend: "Shit or get off the pot!" From her aunt: "One day, she'll run away with another man, and you'll know what a fool you were." From her gay friend: "*I'd* marry her if I weren't gay!" From every woman on planet Earth: "Just like a man: Why buy the cow when you can get the milk for free?" I felt like a stunt man gunning my motorcycle's engine at the edge of the Grand Canyon with everybody yelling, "Come on! You can make it! It's a leap of faith!" But I was frozen.

Over the course of four years, we broke up and got back together dozens of times—all over Our Future. When we weren't talking about a wedding ring, our love was off the charts. But when we did talk about getting married, it shattered. I was in a holding pattern. Whenever I thought about marriage, it was like double-clicking on one side of my brain and opening the independence program, then double-clicking on the other side and getting the same thing! I wanted adventure, and she kept trying to insert marriage/commitment software, and my brain kept rejecting it: *Cannot read disk.*

I needed help, but there was none. My father couldn't com-prehend my predicament because he'd proposed to my mother three weeks after he met her and got married seven weeks later. My buddies were worthless because none could sustain a rela-tionship with a woman for more than a few weeks. And my mar-ried friends all offered the same ambiguous advice: "You just know." *Great! Thanks for the help!* I went to a bookstore and told a saleswoman that I hoped to find a book for "a friend with a major commitment problem." She nodded sympathetically (and muttered under her breath something about her boyfriend). Then she showed me a bunch of psychobabbly commitment books, glossy wedding books, and analytical marriage books. I side-stepped out of the store and nearly broke into a run.

What I needed back then was a book written by a guy for another guy, a lighthearted book with solid tips on how to get through my problem. I wanted advice from a man who had not only conquered his commitment fears but had maintained a sense of adventure in his life and marriage—a book from a man who'd made it to the other side. There was no such book.

I took some hard knocks trying to figure out commitment. After busting through every commitment fear known to mankind, I found peace. One day, after my girlfriend and I had been dating for four years, we were lying in a mud bath at a California spa, and I felt a curi-ous click. I thought, *This is it! This has got to be the woman I'm going to spend my life with!* I would have proposed on the spot, but the rev-elation seemed so strange, so out of character, that I didn't trust myself. Finally, one spring day, while barbecuing under a budding chestnut tree, I proposed. She pulled back and, in a trembling voice, said, "You're kidding, right?" But I wasn't, and she burst into tears and then—to my amazement—I felt ten thousand pounds lighter.

That giddy sensation continued until that great endurance test, Planning the Wedding. As Yogi Berra so notably said, "It ain't over 'til it's over." I needed help there, too—but again, I couldn't find it. And when we returned from our honeymoon, it dawned on me that no guy was going to give me any advice (men don't talk about these things). Once again, there was no book to help.

This is the book I needed back then. It will guide a man through his commitment fears, maintain his commitment through the engagement period and the wedding, and help him keep the zip in his marriage. It's a book about *staying* committed.

The Ring Hurdle feels to many men like leaping through fire. I'm not saying it's easy for a man. I'm not saying it won't be challenging. But I am saying it's worth it. However, it's just not built into our wiring, as it is with so many women.

One foot in front of the other, breath deeply, don't look at the big picture or you'll get dizzy, and know this: Although men resist marriage more than women, we're the ones who enjoy it the most.

But you've got to get over your fears first.

—James Douglas Barron

P.S. I realize that many couples can be emotionally married without tying the knot. For simplicity's sake, I've used all the traditional lingo (*fiancée, husband, wife, marriage*—the words that send shivers up the spine of a commitmentphobic man).

She Wants a Ring

—and I Don't Wanna Change a Thing

TEN GREATEST MOMENTS OF COMMITMENT

1. Falling in love (the easy part of commitment).
2. Saying, "I love you" for the first time—and meaning it.
3. Realizing she's The One.
4. Moving in together—and not freaking out because it feels "too domestic."
5. Understanding that love isn't only about huff-huff, pant-pant, bang-bang sex—and it's OK.
6. Looking at her and suddenly knowing you'll actually propose.
7. Proposing—and feeling lighter than Muhammad Ali on his toes.
8. Telling everyone who had said you'd NEVER DECIDE, "I'm getting married!"
9. Slipping the ring on her finger.
10. Being alone, just the two of you, after the hoopla of the wedding and knowing—divorce rates be damned—you'll make it.

Fighting Your Fears

1. You've fallen for her.

It's not just that women at work are saying, "What's happened to you?" and men are saying, "Wipe that silly grin off your face." Or even that you're calling her phone machine just so you can hear her voice or thinking about the scent of her wrists and neck or God knows where else. You've had all that before—only to discover weeks later that you can't stand the way she picks olives out of her salad.

This is different. You hear an incessant inner voice saying, "She's The One."

2. But she is way ahead of you. She keeps asking, "So, can we talk about our future?"

Gulp. She stares at your hand, and you know she's imagining a ring on it. She sees a baby and gets a look that says, "Get me one of those!" Meanwhile, you're freaking out. You're thinking, *Get me out of this!*

Right now, your idea of commitment is probably limited to not dating anyone else. Her idea of commitment is almost certainly the m-word—marriage.

3. Meanwhile, how do you know for sure if she's The One?

A guy thinks when he finds The One, lightening bolts will flash before his eyes, and fireworks will go off in his head.

Yes, it's a hugely romantic idea that of the billion women on our planet, there's only The One for you. But clearly (and this is Guy Think), there are many lives you could lead. "The One" sounds "out there." (Later, you understand that the woman you choose actually becomes The One over time.)

For now, memorize the ten questions below—so you don't drive your friends nuts with the same, ol' Is-She-The-One? song and dance.

THE 10 QUESTIONS YOU SHOULD ASK YOURSELF

1. Does she bring out the best in me?
2. Do I feel happier when I'm with her or am I merely anxious I'll lose her?
3. Are we best friends or lovers—or both?
4. Are sparks flying? (Enough to get me past the short skirts I'll encounter later?)
5. Am I trying to change her, or is she trying to change me?

6. Can we grow together?
7. Does she have gumption or does she lose it when things get rough?
8. Can I hear myself over everybody else's opinions?
9. Is sex obscuring my vision?
10. Did I get my ya-yas out?

---

4. She's got an internal compass, and you don't. (But is it the right compass?)

She's got True North. You don't. She knows when she's met the right mate. You don't. You feel you're at sea in a boat without a paddle while she stays on course, sailing through the water.

When my then-girlfriend/now-wife wanted to get married, I thought, *Huh? Why would I want to screw up what we've got?* (I was wrong; she was right.) Later, when she wanted to have a baby, I thought, *What? Why would we want to screw up what we've got?* (I was wrong; she was right.) And this pattern has continued throughout my marriage with disturbing regularity.

So, how important is this whole internal-compass thing to a commitment-challenged man? "That's what this whole thing is about," one buddy said. "She's saying, 'I know where our lives are going. You've got to listen to me, honey.'" But you have to do more than just listen; you have to decide if you like the course she's charted. One friend said, "When I couldn't decide on her, I began to focus on where she knew she was going. I decided I didn't want to travel there." Another guy said, "I tried to place my girlfriend in a time-line of my life. Would she have fit in when I was ten? Will she when I'm forty? I decided I would have loved to know her at ten and wanted to see her—and be with her—at forty. I proposed."

Before you get all compassdizzy, remember this: The decision to get serious is a quirky blend of rationality and decision of the heart.

FOR A GUY, THE DECISION TO GET MARRIED IS A SERIES OF EDU- CATED GUESSES. *(For some women—not all—it's intuition.) That's why it's so terrifying for you!*

---

5. The question isn't "Who do you want to be with?" Rather, it's "Who the hell am I?"

Before you can get to the nitty-gritty of deciding if she's right or not, you've got to get your own act together. Otherwise, you'll spend time mentally ripping her to shreds when it's you that needs look- ing at. A classic example was the pompous boyfriend of my friend Judy. He treated her like a Volvo on a hydraulic lift, electrodes and computer hookups monitoring her performance. After several years of constant, unrelenting testing, Judy finally said, "Hey, what about you, Bub?" Not only was he floundering in his career, he was direc- tionless in his life. No introspection. He had an I'm-Better-Than- Everyone-Else attitude. Finally, she dumped him.

If you don't know who you are, try describing yourself in one paragraph. Now try a page. Do you like the man you've summed up?

All this takes some weight off her shoulders and puts it right where it belongs: on yours.

6. *Are you focusing on her "baggage"?*

Never say, "She's OK, but she's got baggage." Women hate hearing about your dislike of their "baggage" not only because it implies that you, Your Lordliness, haveth no baggage, but because they seem to understand that love is, in the immortal baritone of Rocky, about *fillin' in gaps. . . .*

7. *Who were you looking for, anyway?*

Try this simple exercise: Write down who you think you were looking for. Start with Guy Stuff: her looks, your sex life, how she makes you feel. Then move on to Social Stuff: religion, education, family background, social upbringing, career. Now get on to Tough Stuff: her vision of your future together, kids, travel, home.

Perhaps the woman you love doesn't match the requirements you thought you needed in a woman. I know I went through my dating years looking for a Prescribed Woman. The curious thing is, I'd met her on numerous occasions—and she never flipped my switch. She was too aggressive for my taste, too athletic, too proper, too whatever.

Maybe you're like me, and your subconscious nudged you to find your opposite. My opposite was lighter and more carefree, not as burdened by the big stuff in life. She'd let herself go more in her early years, didn't care about grades, flunked a few things without losing sleep, didn't care what others thought. She was quicker than me, but less of a worker. I felt I needed this type of woman, just as she would need me. Some relationships are about counterbalance, and maybe yours falls into that category, too.

Remember: Everything can't be scripted. Leave room for the unexpected.

8. The question is not "Can you live without her?"

The question is "Is she too good to let go?"

9. How do you know you won't fall harder for the woman around the corner?

Well, you don't. But isn't all of life like that? If you didn't make a move out of fear that something better was waiting, you'd be paralyzed.

Reality check: You will be tempted by other women because the world is filled with amazing women. But you'll never know what it would be like because you're not going to go there. Period. Would another woman be better than the one you have? Who knows?

If you try to be certain about everything, you'll end up with nothing.

10. Listen to your gut.

The problem is, most guys have trouble telling which part of their anatomy is talking: The Gut, The Brain, or The Penis. Your gut talks in a mumbled, soft whisper, and your natural inclination is to say, "I can't hear you! Next!" Your brain talks in a stern, paternal, librarian tone, and your inclination is to say, "Boring! Next!" And your penis shrieks at you day and night, "Let's P-A-R-T-Y!" Your inclination is to say, "Sure. Did you say blonde, brunette, or redhead?"

Try this simple exercise. Think back to when you met your girlfriend. Write down your first reaction. There was a soft voice that said, yes or no. If you're honest with yourself, you'll realize you heard that voice and probably shoved it away. Big mistake.

Now try to remember if you had some strong gut reactions in later months or years. One buddy said, "After four torturous years,

I finally found my gut on two occasions. Both times, it felt like an out-of-body experience. It was as if I were watching a movie. I thought, *Yes, this is a wonderful woman. But no, this is not the woman you are supposed to spend the rest of your life with.* It was as if my gut yelled, 'OK! Here it is! I'm telling you the answer! If you spend the rest of your life with this woman, you will not become the person you want to be!' "

As a general rule, be careful not to listen too closely to your brain. It can and will engage in tedious, Senate-like debates, often playing devil's advocate just for the sport of it. (The result: Everyone is fast asleep.) Get back to your gut. It's like going for the final shot in basketball. Coach diagrams a play, you learn it. Then you have to forget it so when you can get the ball, you can use your gut. Same thing, reacting to a woman. Forget all the diagrams your mind has constructed. She's right or she's wrong. React.

11. Know two important rules: (1) Not being able to say yes is the same as saying no, and (2) don't beat yourself up for not coming up with the answer.

"It's like in a trial," said my friend Daryl, a lawyer. "You don't have to prove that the person is innocent. You have to prove that the person is guilty beyond a reasonable doubt. Likewise, when I was trying to decide on Linda, I couldn't decide beyond a reasonable doubt that she was right for me. There was nothing wrong with her. We made each other happy. We were attracted to each other, had a good sex life, and had a good time together. But I couldn't get past my doubts. I finally took two weeks off from work, stared at the ceiling, and *considered*. It was like Chinese water torture; I went totally out of my mind. A good buddy, who's been married a dozen years, finally said, 'Hey, you can't decide? You're *this* whacked out? Working a chain gang would be heaven compared to what you've got? That means no.'

"He was right. Later, I met a woman who I could prove beyond a reasonable doubt was right for me."

12. *Don't let her pursue you.*

You love being pursed for about two milliseconds; then you resent it. There's a little problem here. With your indecision, you've become the fox, and she's become the hound. You're panting and winded while she's sprinting after you, yelling "Why are you running? I just want to talk about *Us!*"

The more she pushes you, the less chance that you'll ask her to marry you. Why? Men hate being pressured. One guy told me that after years of dating, he'd finally met the woman he would marry. "I was totally, completely, absolutely in love," he said. "She was perfect. But then on our second date, we were playing tennis in a remote spot and everything changed. I was shining my car headlights over the court since it had gotten dark and the court had no lights. I went to retrieve the tennis balls in the corner. When I turned, she had stripped off all her clothes. My heart sank. Suddenly, *she was after me.* I thought, *What does she want from me? If she would do this for me, she would have done it for other men before me. And she might do it for other men after me.*" The relationship never recovered.

Sure, half the fun of falling in love is turning the rules upside down. In fact, falling in love *is* turning the rules upside-down. But if you're like most guys, you still need to feel you're doing the chasing, and not the one being chased.

HER 6 GREATEST FEARS ABOUT STAYING WITH YOU WHILE YOU'RE MAKING UP YOUR MIND

1. You'll waste her best years and then dump her for a younger woman with a taut face and bouncy buns.
2. She'll help you forge a career, and another woman will get all the perks.
3. Every girlfriend of hers will get married and have babies while she waits for you to make up your mind.
4. She'll pass up a guy who worships her and has a rock the size of a Quarter Pounder awaiting her finger.
5. You'll never decide.
6. You'll decide, engagement will be heaven, and then you'll *undecide* before the wedding.

13. If pairing off permanently is so natural, how come it seems so repellent?

Well, think of the questions that have ricocheted through the minds, souls, and groins of every man who's ever lived: On a planet populated by millions of gorgeous females, is it really possible to limit yourself to one? Won't sex with your woman—which has so far sizzled like an egg on Alabama asphalt in August—eventually become so dull she'll say, "OK, but only if it's quick. I've got a 7:15 breakfast meeting"? Why should you marry when half the married couples you know are ready to rip each other's heads off (or let their lawyers do the decapitations for them)—and the other half are divorced? Or when the cool married couples (whom everyone you know said, "See? It can be done,") are now on the rocks? And will she love you after you're wider than you are tall, with more hair on your back than on your head? Won't farting, belching, nosepicking and buttscratching (not to mention childbirth) kill off what's left of lust?

No. Here's something nobody has bothered to explain to men: Once you're married to a woman, you're forever the guy who made the over-the-shoulder catch into deep center field. She's forever the young woman wading in the surf at sunset to watch hermit crabs scamper. There's a secret knowledge you and she carry of when you two were young, wild, and passionate. Nobody else owns that—and nobody can take it away.

10 THINGS A MAN FEARS MOST ABOUT MARRIAGE

1. The life sentence: "For better or worse." (*Clank! Cell door shut!*)
2. Giving up that dream of tasting the fruits of all nations (flitting from woman to woman in a glorious bath of love and lust).

3. The "What If?" complex (as in, *What if I fall even more in love with another woman?*).
4. Divorce (as in betting on a loser).
5. Replicating your parents' failed marriage. (Or replicating your parents' happy marriage—and one day calling your wife "Angel," "Sugarplum," or "Darl.")
6. Surrendering your post as president and CEO of the firm Fun. Then having to answer to a board of directors in a firm called Compromise, fully knowing every decision can come under kill-joy scrutiny.
7. Becoming an active member in the Tamed Husband fraternity.
8. The Blah Life (boredom, overfamiliarity, and routine).
9. Surrendering quiet, control, space, privacy, watching ESPN all night, poker and suds with the guys, cigar breath, stinky sneakers . . .
10. Giving up Erotic Break-the-Guest-Room-Fold-Out-Couch Sex for Regulated You-Do-This, I-Do-That, Now-Let's-Sleep Sex.

---

14. But don't go full speed ahead if you don't know where you're going.

Sometimes a guy who is secretly afraid of commitment hops into a relationship as if it were a cigarette boat in a James Bond flick: He twists the throttle, romances the hell out of her, and pretends that he and she are zooming off toward Forever Land. He knows there's a leak in the fuel tank and the boat's likely to explode into smithereens at any moment, but he refuses to slow down. Instead, he hopes she'll notice the message in the boat's wake: *All this romancing is a big lie!* But many women are commitment starved and enjoy the wild ride—until you slam into the breakwall of your unacknowledged commitment fears and the relationship sinks.

Don't let your insecurity drive you into Coverup Mode. Let your relationship build day by day. No grand pronouncements. No plane tickets to Hawaii after Week One. No talk about buying a '66 Ford convertible and driving across the country with her. No staring at pups in the pet store window and muttering how you envision a new home with a yard and a dog with a bone. Maybe you want marriage in your future, and maybe you think you *ought* to be ready, but don't try to convince yourself by convincing her.

---

6 THINGS YOU'LL SAY THAT MAKE HER BELIEVE YOU'LL BE TOGETHER FOREVER (AND WILL GET YOU IN TROUBLE IF YOU DON'T FOLLOW THROUGH)

1. "I can't live without you."
2. "You make me feel complete."
3. "I feel like I've known you my whole life."
4. "I can't remember what my life was like before we were together."
5. "I've never felt so comfortable with anyone before."
6. "I'm going to take care of you from now on."

---

15. Don't say, "I love you, but . . ."

Her heart skips a beat as you declare your love—and then you muck up the whole thing by adding, "but."

To women, there are no "buts" in love. Love is an absolute. By definition, it contradicts everything in reality: There are no rules, no boundaries, no sense of time, order, or status.

The problem is, the man who finds another clause after "I love you" can never finish the sentence correctly. It's that simple. Whatever qualifiers, contexts, stipulations, or riders he tags on, he comes off as the Big Loser.

Check out these bungled declarations:

The Classic: "I love you, but . . . I need a little more time."

The Astronaut: "I love you, but . . . I need some space."

The Contradiction: "I love you, but . . . I'm not *in love* with you."

The Too-Early Excuse: "I love you, but . . . I wish I'd met you five years from now."

The Too-Late Excuse: "I love you, but . . . I wish I'd met you five years ago."

The Workaholic Excuse: "I love you, but . . . my career isn't there yet."

The Poetic Excuse: "I love you, but . . . ours is true love and marriage is ordinary love."

The Klutz Excuse: "I love you, but . . . I'd only wreck it."

The Testosterone Excuse: "I love you, but . . . I'm a man, and there are women to meet and dates to be had, dancers to dance on my lap, yet-unknown women to whisper in my ear, 'Take me, now,' etc. etc."

In the end, either she won't hear the explanation. Or it will just trigger the fight that immediately follows.

16. Be Careful: Everything you say may be interpreted as "He's afraid of commitment."

After you've had The Commitment Discussion countless times, both of you have a hard time discussing anything else. (The Commitment Discussion centers on whether or not you'll marry her; "anything else" might include your concerns about money, religion, goals, and so on.) "It's like those bad subtitles on a foreign film," my friend Daryl said. "Someone talks on and on and *on*, and finally there's a two word subtitle. Similarly, I would talk on and on and on, and what she'd hear was 'He's afraid of commitment.' I had to say, 'Wait a minute. You're not listening!'"

There's also a point when it seems that you and she can't have fun without it being proof that You Are the Ideal Couple, which equals It's Time to Tie the Knot. "After a while, all roads led to the same thing," one guy said. "We'd have fun, and she'd say, 'See? What are you waiting for?' We'd have a bad time, and she'd say, 'See? This wouldn't have happened if we were married.' I had to tell her that my fear of commitment was *not* responsible for everything!"

FOR MEN, "COMMIT" IS AN UGLY WORD. You're thinking of these dictionary definitions: "To place officially in confinement or custody" and "Official consignment, as to a prison or mental hospital."

She skips to another meaning: "To pledge oneself . . . entrust and confide." How is it that her perspective is so different?

17. Define your fear of commitment.

What makes commitment fear so vexing for your partner is that you're equally afraid of forever in its various forms. Losing her *is* forever. Committing to her *is* forever.

If you come on like gangbusters—wine and dine her and carry on like a lunatic about love, kids, and her gorgeous green eyes—and the next instant you think about the woman in the twitching jeans walking ten feet in front of you (you don't know her—and that's the point), you've got a fear of commitment.

If you invite your girlfriend to the company's Christmas party and then renege at the last moment, claiming you've got a cold and you're hitting the hay early—when, in reality, you met a woman with a great smile, great hips, a great walk that afternoon and asked *her* to the party—you've got a fear of commitment.

If you break up with your girlfriend, and she accepts the breakup, saying, "OK, I'll get on with my life. In fact, I'm leaving on Monday to go skiing in Jackson Hole," and then you bombard her with an avalanche of flowers, E-mail messages, phone calls, invitations to dinner, and pleas to her friends, begging her to come back—and she does. Then the instant you've got her, you want to run away—you've got a fear of commitment.

If you're stalling about moving in together—even though your girlfriend of one year has to go home every night at midnight to walk her weak-bladdered basset hound, and you've promised her marriage "one day," but you just can't pull the trigger, even on naming the date—you've got a fear of commitment.

You want it all. Closeness and distance at the same time.

Well, it just won't work out that way.

SO WHY DON'T YOU WANNA CHANGE A THING? You're juggling the male desire to have sex with every beautiful babe who squiggles past your line of vision and your need for complete commitment to one woman.

There is good news and bad news. Bad news first: Your attraction to other woman will never go totally away (which means you'll always be slightly crazed). Now the good news: It's normal. You can live and thrive within your wild mind. You can toss it all together into the salad you call Life with Wife.

If this fight ever goes away completely, you'd better check your pulse.

---

18. Are you terrified of love the instant it becomes reciprocal?

My friend Gina was nearly driven nuts when her boyfriend Karl upped the ante by saying, "I never want to leave you," "I love you forever," "I want you to be the mother of my children," "Let's get married—someday soon," and "Move out to Colorado with me. Please. Now. You must" (all this after two weeks).

Gina quit her job, packed her bags, moved halfway across the continent—and nearly the instant she got there, Karl became another person: cold, indifferent, incapable of helping her find a new job. When she moved out, he barely raised a stir.

Flash forward two years. Gina bumped into Karl at a party. He begged for forgiveness, they fell wildly in love again, he pleaded that they move in together (again, after only two weeks). "I'm so happy in northern California! You've got to live with me! It will be perfect this time! I won't let you down!"

"Every cell in my body told me not to do it, but I didn't listen," she said. She headed west and—almost before she could say, "God-damn-am-I-stupid!"—he froze, and she packed her bags and moved out again.

OK, you may not be as afflicted as Karl. Still, the lesson here is Crazy Glue your tongue to the roof of your mouth if you think you're about to make promises you won't keep. ("I meant it when I said it," will not hold up in the courtroom of her mind.)

19. Step up your behavior if she's a single mom.

You may feel that you get no slack: You've got to decide if you want to jump from being a single man to being a father without having time to adjust during the pregnancy. You're suspicious of the way she slowly releases the truth about her past (her husband and the divorce) and her present (her child or children). And you're obviously inheriting some problems you didn't create.

But pushing those considerations to the side, you've got to operate on a higher level of conduct than those of us commitmentphobes who are dating nonmothers. Single moms—and their children—deserve a whole different set of behavior. Kid gloves. Kindness. Don't say anything you don't mean. Don't move in with her unless you've considered the damage you'll do to her kids when you move out.

My friend Bev was thirty years old, recently divorced, and a single mother with a two-year-old girl when she started dating her now-husband. "Before I even allowed him into my home, I said, 'I can't have you waltzing in and out of my life. I've got a precious daughter who comes first.' He promised to respect that. Then the first time he was over (after three months of dating), he came into the kitchen and said, 'Your daughter just called me Daddy.' I said, 'You all right with that?' He just smiled and hugged me, and I kinda knew it would all work out." (They've now been married nine years and have a second daughter.)

Flipside: You may become unbelievably attached to a single mother's kids—and breaking up will be debilitating not only to the kids, but to you. "I've never been married," said my pal Adam, "but I feel like I've lost two kids. Even four years later, even though Pam's re-married, I keep a photo of her kids in my wallet at all times. My heart's broken."

Marrying a single mom may even be an incentive, as it was for Bev's husband, Dan, and for my friend Nick. "I felt I was getting a package deal," Nick said. "It was great. I suddenly had a kid. I had a wife. Instant family."

20. Beware of your self-imposed Ideal Marriage Age.
Every guy picks an age when he envisions being married. Then he starts dating, and the Ideal Marriage Age moves back, and back and back. Then, if he turns forty, he realizes he's outlived that date and gets antsy.

It's easy to run amuck if you let your Ideal Marriage Age dictate when you'll marry. My pal Ivan's dad was married at twenty-one. He said, "It's weird to admit, but I felt over the hill at twenty-two. So, I married the wrong woman just to stay on schedule and was divorced three years later. A big part of my hang-up on getting married young had to do with my parents' definition of 'normalcy.' My advice to guys is, *Don't get married to please your parents.*"

My magic number was thirty-five. I figured that by then, I'd have enough of a chance to get my ya-yas out. The trouble was, I met the woman who would become my bride when I was twenty-seven. Four years later, I proposed. I griped to buddies that I was still, by New York City standards, a social embryo. Women didn't even start taking me seriously until I was twenty-six! I was a grape picked before my time! But I had found the right woman—and that made it the right time.

21. Be honest with her.

Stress that you're not trying to hurt her and that what bothers you most is that you *are* hurting her. But remind her that the pressure is slowly killing you—and you're afraid of letting go of the relationship just so the pressure may ease (it won't). Tell her that you want to get through it together.

Most of the guys I know who've been plagued by this indecision get nuts over their fear of failure. My friend Steve said, "No matter how much I was succeeding in every other aspect of my life (work, money, home), I woke up each day, looked in the mirror, and said, 'You can't get it together! You're indecisive! You wobble!' I wanted to run from her so I could run from the failure."

My friend Daryl said, "Since I'd been in this situation three times before, I found myself comparing my feelings and worrying about how I'd feel if I failed again. It all seemed familiar."

Your honesty may prompt hers. She may say, "You're never going to know for sure. If you think I'm 100 percent certain inside, you're wrong. But I do believe in our future together, and I know we've got a limited time to lock into it."

22. Tell her you understand what she's going through.

Really, you shouldn't have to try hard to empathize with her situation. She's invested a lot of herself in a relationship that may end before you make up your mind. That can't be easy. Take a look around, and you'll see everyone harping and haranguing her about how difficult you are, what a jerk you are, and about how decision impaired you are.

Will any of this cut you any slack? Probably not. But at least you're showing her that you can look beyond your own hang-ups and see her perspective, too.

23. The moment will come (if it hasn't already) when she can't stay with you one more goddamned second if you don't promise that you'll some day, somehow, get married.

You're flying back from the perfect vacation, sipping wine, her head resting on your shoulder, when everything changes. You've had your week of bliss: lolling on a beach, running naked in the waves, eating grilled fish under a thatched-roof cabana, and gazing into the shifting blue and green waters.

But all this paradise was an illusion. Trouble has been brewing. Now that you're heading home, you feel it coming: The Talk. Although you'd agreed to a cease-fire from airport to airport, she simply can't resist. So, pushing her lips to your ear, she whispers warmly, "I've never been happier."

"Neither have I," you say cheerily, taking a sudden interest in the headphones.

"What could be better?" she asks, circling her finger on your chest in what seems to be the shape of a wedding band.

You feel suddenly hot, claustrophobic. You twist the air vent. The flow seems anemic. You have a sudden desire to try parachuting.

She stares into your eyes. "You *are* getting closer, right? You know I can't wait forever," she says.

You kiss her forehead, then resort to one of your pat lines: "I need just a bit more time." "I'm almost there." "I really want to, but I can't yet." (Then you go back to examining the head phones.)

She sits bolt upright and, in no particular order, reels off phrase after dreaded phrase, the ones that have been delivered from womankind to mankind for millennia: "You think anything could be better?" "What are you looking for, PERFECTION?" "You're wasting my best years!" "I've got to know about *Us*." "Everybody wants to know why the hell I stay with someone who can't decide!"

You probably won't end up in the same cab back from the airport. And while you watch her zoom off in a taxi, you'll think, *Do I have a commitment problem? Is she just not The One? If she hadn't forced the issue, would I have decided by now? Or, am I totally schizo?*

Welcome to commitment hell.

9 INDICATIONS THAT YOU'RE IN A HOLDING PATTERN

1. You chase, nab, and discard women the way a day-trader goes in and out of tech stocks.
2. Women tell you, "Either you shut down when things get emotional or you have no emotions."
3. You run your relationships the way Steinbrenner does the Yankees: with an iron fist.
4. You find troubled women, then vow to change them. (When they're changed, you drop them, or they hop into a banged-up Chevy with a slimy, tattoo-covered ex-con and drive away.)
5. You're addicted to distance. (She lives in Milan. You live in Los Angeles. You like having only twenty minutes of feasible telephone time to connect while one of you isn't asleep or cheating on the other.)
6. You have a history of finding "cheatin' women." (Afterwards, you find solace in the words of gravel-voiced country singers with hangdog faces.)
7. You're into "playing house" with women—knowing you'll never end up at the altar.
8. After being dumped by a woman, you eat nothing but Spam slathered with mustard for the ensuing two years—but refuse to see a shrink.
9. You don't have the heart to end relationships. Instead, you say to yourself, "If I have to get married, I could always get divorced."

24. Ask yourself, How much of this is narcissism?

Are you the kind of guy who takes trophy girlfriends to public places so everyone will marvel? Are you really worried that friends don't find her gorgeous? That people won't think you're the-next-George-Clooney if you're with her? At restaurants, do you sit facing the mirror (or reflective glass) so you can admire the slick way you throw your head back when you laugh?

If you're hung up on these things, you're not ready.

25. How much of this is Pecker Power Proving?

For some guys: none. For others: some. For yet others: a ton (hell—all of it!).

One guy told me, "When I met the woman who is now my wife, all I could think was, *I wonder what she looks like naked.* The thought stuck in my brain until we had sex (later that night). And from that moment on, all I could think was, *She loves me because I'm such a great lover.* We had sex constantly and got married six months later.

"But one day, she stopped wanting to have sex so much. At first, it was three times a week. Then once a week. Then once every two weeks. Then once a month. Then all I could think was, *She doesn't love the way I make love to her any more.*"

Here's the rule: Don't marry her if it's only about Pecker Power Proving. Because when the sex slows, another woman will shoot you that *Come Prove Your Pecker Power to Me* look. If that's how you define yourself as a guy, you're in trouble.

P.S. So what's the deal with Pecker Power Proving? For some

guys, it's a question of looking at their penis, then a ruler, and asking, "Is the ruler Half Empty or Half Full?" (Then trying, as often as possible, to prove they can satisfy a woman.) For others, it's about keeping score. For others, it's about . . . whatever. Don't go there!

BEWARE OF THE "CINDY" SYNDROME. ("IF CINDY CRAWFORD BREAKS UP WITH HER HUSBAND, I STILL HAVE A CHANCE.") While you obsess over Cindy (or a variation of Cindy), you're missing out on real relationships.

---

26. Fantasy and reality are different.

Unfortunately, most guys never learn this simple truth—or they learn it the hard way.

I interviewed a guy who has indulged every fantasy. He'd done twosomes, threesomes, foursomes (in all combinations of male-to-female and female-to-male), slept with his girlfriend's best friend and allowed his girlfriend to sleep with his best friend. "It's not what you'd expect it to be," he told me. "You've pictured all this stuff in your head since you were thirteen, but now your head gets in the act. There's a distance you can't avoid. Somehow, it's more immediate when it's *just* in your head."

Fantasies are great because they have no consequences. Go ahead: Travel with your fantasies. Keep them in your head—and, much later, share them with the woman you love.

•   •   •

27. Are you afraid of never watching another woman undress for you again?

Forget Kilimanjaro at sunrise; there's no greater sight in all nature than a beautiful woman shedding her clothes for you for the very first time. She's teasing you as she tugs at the buttons. She's slipping her blouse past her shoulders. She's loosening her bra. She's kicking her panties at you. (Enough said . . . and wipe that drool off the page.)

You guess that by the time you've seen the woman you love naked a thousand times, you won't even raise your eyes while you're peeing into the toilet and she's steaming up the shower. Or you wonder how you'll react when your wife, clad in long johns, is bedridden with the flu and pyramids of used tissues rise from the bed.

And you've got to wonder if she'll do anything but laugh when you rip off your T-shirt, flex your flabby abs, and deliver that Let's Get Down Tonight look.

You say to yourself, *This isn't what I want! She doesn't want it either! Resisting commitment is a gift to her, too!*

Will you ever be as breathless as when you first touched her breasts? No. But nobody bothers to assure guys that when you first meet a woman, it's like picking up a guitar for the first time; later, you're like Hendrix playing his Strat (wah-wah pedal and all).

28. When the crazy, early days go, the show's not over.

Ah . . . falling in love. Your blood is boiling with hormones and natural chemicals. You're like a junkie: *more, more!*

But when the natural high goes, you discover what you're

made of as a couple, because your relationship will be tied to the laws of normal life. It's like midnight on the Fourth of July; when the fireworks are over; it's time to go home.

Yeah, fireworks are fine—but they're also loud and bright; you'd be blind and deaf if they continued indefinitely. Marriage is more subtle and rewarding than that.

29. Married sex can be hot sex. It can be explosive sex. It can be even better than early sex.

There's a type of sex that every guy loves: walk-in-the-door-rip-off-the-clothes-trip-over-the-coffee-table-do-it-on-the-floor sex. Unfortunately, men believe that when that type of sex dies, there's nothing to replace it.

Wrong. Your sex life with one woman goes through cycles, which include coming back to the walk-in-the-door-etc type. Next comes Let's-Play-with-All-Five-Senses sex. Extremely erotic stuff. Following that is Total-Knowing-Each-Other sex. That's when you know every thought in her head, every dream, every wish. After that comes Lemme-Try-This-Out sex. That's when you're so loving, trusting and understanding that you're allowed to live out each other's fantasies—on each other. Finally, there's Cosmic Sex. That's when suddenly and without warning, you're making love and you touch something beyond human comprehension. You see her as a little girl and an older woman all at once. The next instant you feel you're a couple of kids playing with mud pies, your body *is* hers, and there is no rest of the world.

We're all conditioned by advertising to think that young people screw better. Well, they don't. As everyone knows, you can't sustain pedal-to-the-metal sex with one person forever. You've got to get to the next stage and the ones beyond that.

And guess what: After you've had Cosmic Sex, you'll need a breather. After a week or two, you'll start the cycle again.

DON'T TALK LIKE AN ANIMAL BEHAVIORIST WHEN YOU DISCUSS MONOGAMY. My friend Hal is always citing the sexual habits of rodents, fish, and fowl when he argues for polygamy. He's always expounding on the "male need to perpetuate the species." Women roll their eyes.

---

30. Ask yourself, How much of this is just a fear of getting older?

You're at a restaurant with your girlfriend when a bunch of fifty-something couples are seated at the next table. They seem about as unappealing as five-day-old mashed potatoes. Clearly, you think, kids have knocked them smack-dab into neuterland. They're talking about renovation nightmares and 401ks and pink drinks with little umbrellas on beach vacations, and they're laughing, chortling, snorting at . . . whatever. You whisper to your girlfriend, "These folks need to get laid." She says, "You're terrified of getting old, aren't you?"

You excuse yourself and dash to the john. Staring into the mirror at your hairline, you think, *She's right.*

For lots of single guys, marriage seems like the nail poised on the coffin lid. So keep this in mind: The eternal bachelor who's a regular at a bar, meets and beds chicks half his age, dies younger than the committed, married man. And what happens to the pickup artist when he's beyond his prime? You see these guys in their later years, paunchy and bald, stirring sugar into their coffee at a ratty diner.

31. She will hate when you say, "I just need some space."

She wants a space with two people in it. A comfy, cuddly space.

You want the high plains with John Lennon, Muddy Waters, and Kurt Cobain singing "I Am a Walrus" from the clouds. Mustangs here. Buffalo there.

"Whenever my boyfriend talked about space," one woman said, "I'd reply, 'Oh, go work at NASA!'"

Try to remind her that the need for space is a huge part of marriage, too. (Nobody likes to be shrinkwrapped; we would suffocate.) But men are somewhat different in this regard: We need to venture out into the world and then settle back into a *shared* space. When men talk about the need for space, we mean that we don't want constant intimacy. We don't want to be shackled, or we feel invaded.

Instead of begging for more space, be more specific. Tell her where you're going and when you'll be back. With time, she'll get accustomed to your need to go out into the world and boomerang back. (She'll probably never see it as your most endearing quality, though.)

32. Consider a break.

When all you do is fight (you're not going to propose, and she's not going to wait), a break can be the best medicine.

One friend said, "A lot of guys have the same fear: If we take a break, she'll go out with another man." What he's really saying is, *Most men are worried she'll get the fuck of her life.* Then, when you come scampering back, she'll say, "I don't need you anymore. Meet Jack. He subsidized his own Everest climb—and his penis arrived at the summit ten seconds before his torso." (Then, you'll lay on the shrink's couch the rest of your life.)

How long a break do you need? Two weeks? A month? Two months? Or, as one friend said, "Try a season." (But that's only if you've been together way too long and still can't decide.) Will you date other people? Agree on the rules and then stick to them (as best you can).

Good news: After a break, you may fall in love *more* absolutely (that means, without the barracks you have formerly constructed). You see things more clearly, and you tie the knot.

33. You should tell her exactly how much time you think you need.

While you're deciding, her looks are fading (at least in her mind). Your sperm count could still be good at sixty, seventy, or maybe eighty (don't bet the house on eighty), but she's got a finite number of eggs and a shorter cutoff date for getting pregnant. Be realistic: If your girlfriend is in her late thirties and hopes to have a baby, you've got less time to decide (and less married time before you try to start a family). These are important considerations.

So, how much time should it take to make your decision? (As much as she'll give you plus two months.) Instead, circle a date on the calendar. Make your own ultimatum. Say, "If we can't decide in six months, don't you think it's better that we call it quits?" She'll probably agree.

Tough medicine. But better than the nowhereland you've created.

---

6 RESPONSES THAT SHE REALLY DOESN'T WANT TO HEAR WHEN SHE ASKS, "WHEN WILL YOU BE READY?"

1. "How much time do I have?"
2. "I wish I knew."
3. "Is this an ultimatum?"
4. "Can I get back to you on this?"
5. "This isn't about you. It's about me."
6. "What's your definition of 'sex with another woman'?"

---

34. *You can learn a lot from your parents' marriage.*
My friend Patrick's parents got divorced when he was eight (they were separated when he was six). But after years of marriage and divorce, marriage and divorce (and refusing to speak to one another), his parents met again at a family funeral and were clearly—to Patrick's eyes—still wildly in love. This revelation was both consoling (he always had hoped his parents still loved one another) and extraordinarily tragic (they blew it by not getting through the tough times). "I learned how *not* to be married from my parents.

When things got difficult in my own marriage, I knew not to run away. The next marriage and the one after that wouldn't be any better—and might be a lot worse."

I heard the same stuff repeatedly from friends: "I learned every possible thing *not* to do in marriage." And "My parents had a horrible marriage. The night before they were going to marry, my mother went to her father and said, 'I don't love him.' He replied, 'We're having one hundred fifty people for a barbeque tomorrow. You're going to marry him.' It took my mother eighteen years to get out of the wrong marriage." And "I watched my parents live in mutual hate for their entire lives. Before I could face marriage, I had to convince myself I could create a marriage not based on their rules."

Consider yourself lucky if you admire your parents' marriage. Otherwise, learn in reverse. Tell her what qualities you refuse to replicate. Then stick to it.

35. Remember that security can set you free.

With someone behind you, supporting you, believing in your dream as you do, you may just take a leap you wouldn't dare alone. Start that company. Invent that product. Paint that painting. You can be liberated—not frozen—by marriage because you have a place to rest at the end of the day.

"After we got married," my friend Ken told me, "my wife said, 'Take a shot at your dream.' Then, for one year, she supported me with her income while I set up my business."

You can also divide and conquer. When my friend Phil got married, he asked his wife if she'd mind telling him if there was anything important to read in the newspaper (she didn't mind;

there was usually nothing vital), so he could finally get around to reading the complete works of Shakespeare.

No, these are not reasons to get married. But they are benefits that you won't know until you take the leap.

36. Remember that security can set you free, too.
Ask her to close her eyes and dream *her* dream. (Some of her dreams may be to pursue interests, like drawing or dancing, that she gave up as a kid—under the banner of Growing Up.) Perhaps you don't need two incomes. You can suggest that she quit her job.

Make her dream come true, and you're bound forever.

37. Control your attacks of Domesticity Claustrophobia.
She cooks you a chicken dinner. She sets out candles. And wine. And staring into your eyes, says, "Doesn't this feel . . . *won-der-ful?*"

You squeak, "Y-yes."

Rather than sit down for the meal, you grab the horn and call a buddy. He tells you about a beer party with your buddies. You scarf down the meal and head out the door, leaving her muttering, "I don't deserve this."

(Or you don't go to the party but pull away, hoping she won't notice in the ensuing weeks that you've stopped making love, bringing flowers, and buying her gifts.)

The rule is: *The more you pull back, the more she wants you,* which sets up her response of tugging you closer. Your fear of intimacy kicks her into high gear.

Ask yourself, *Why am I feeling claustrophobic?* Usually, it's because staring into the poultry on your table, you see suits with penitentiary stripes, a house with a yard, a subscription to the symphony, and maybe even orthodontia for the kids and college tuition bills. Stop yourself from zooming off into the unknown. Don't let your fears of the future wreck what you've got.

GUESS WHAT: SHE WANTS DIFFERENT THINGS FROM THE RELATION-SHIP. The cliché is this: She's after safety, security, comfort, companionship, understanding, and someone to calm her when she freaks out. You're after sex, someone to make you feel big and important, and someone to listen to you.

But that's a gross simplification. Contrary to popular opinion, men thrive on the comfort and security of marriage. In fact, we sometimes get so addicted that we turn into total homebodies. Look at the stats and you'll see that it's married men who are the most contented (more than single men, married women, and single women).

---

38. She's eager to bring out the "real you": a guy who can cry and laugh and hug and kiss and play footsie.

No wonder you're nervous.

She believes that your stereotypical male behavior is a product of having had an uncaring father (then having adopted Clint Eastwood, Arnold Schwartzenegger, Bruce Lee, or early-Bruce Willis as a mock-surrogate dad) and of society's demand that a *real man* (the type who opens a can of chili with his teeth, grrrrr) shows no emotions. She cringes when one of your male friends says, "How's business?" (instead of "How are you?") and you reply, "Business is great!" (instead of "I'm OK . . . but my dad has been in and out of doctors' offices all week and I'm worried.").

Why evolve in this direction? Because you're changing each other for the better; that's what a relationship is about!

39. No, you're not on a tell-all talk show.
Not to discourage getting things out in the open . . . but *everything?*

You're having a quiet drink at a quiet place when one of you decides the time is right to spill the beans. "My mother is an alcoholic," she says. "My dad is, too," you reply. "My mother accidentally burned the house down when she fell asleep with a lit cigarette," she counters. "My father lost his money in the stock market and sat on the couch for three years with a tortilla chip glued to his lower lip, and I've never overcome the fear of abandonment," you say. "I'm not comfortable with my breasts," she says. You say, "I always wanted to be John Holmes." ("He's dead," she says. "Still . . ." you say.) OK, weird stuff happens and strange thoughts occur to everyone—but your relationship is not a toxic waste site, and your lover is *not* your therapist.

There's a timetable for absolving yourself of every sad story—not too soon, not all at once, but before engagement and marriage. However, all of us have an ozone layer that protects us. You need to retain a little mystery for yourself and the woman you love.

40. Get your terminology straight: She's your G-I-R-L-F-R-I-E-N-D.

One female friend said, "After eight months, Tom still couldn't call me his 'girlfriend.' I'd seen him five nights a week. We were intimate. We celebrated holidays together. I'd met (and put up with) his parents. I helped him through tough spells with his boss and work and health. And he literally couldn't verbalize 'girlfriend.' "

Another friend told me that one night, when she was lying in bed with her boyfriend, he tipped his wine glass to hers and toasted, "I've had a great time hanging out with you." She bolted upright, pulled the covers over her, and said, "You think we've been 'hanging out?!' Oh, my God! Oh, so that's what we've been doing?!" Within minutes, she had her clothes on and stormed out the door. "It was raining buckets, and he lived in a not-so-great part of town. I didn't have an umbrella. I was seething. When I got home, I stood by the phone, just waiting. *I know he's going to call.* When he didn't, I thought: This is O-V-E-R." And it was.

Here's the point: *Guy talk doesn't translate to women.* When you tell another guy you "had a great time hanging out," it's tantamount to being blood brothers. To a woman, it means nothing.

41. Introduce her to your friends.

You've probably been neglecting your old friends. They'll ask why. You don't have the heart to say, "Know what? You guys just can't compete." (But it's the truth.)

One day, the huff-huff, pant-pant, bang-bang, crazy early days of romance wane. Look out. You want your friends and you want her. But, you sequester her from your friends. There's an odd sort of male logic operating here: It may be you're afraid she will run off with one of your buddies. My friend Eric explained the phenomenon: "She was so sexy, and none of them had girl-friends. I was insecure. I thought she'd dump me for one friend who's six-four, has a cool business, travels all over the world, and had just broken up with his girlfriend. All paranoia—all in my mind." His girlfriend said, "Whenever he was with his friends, I felt he wanted to shove me in a closet and toss the key. It was so offensive."

Or maybe you're keeping her away from your group so they won't think it's a serious relationship when you're not sure. Including her would be putting a brand on you: *"I'm Taken! Out of Circulation!"* (And maybe you feel you're not ready for other women to stay away.)

If you're in the relationship, be *in* the relationship. Involve her with your friends, challenge your paranoia, and let people think what they will.

BUT ARE YOU, IN FACT, A DECISION INVALID? I know I was.

Hell, I couldn't buy anything without returning it a few times (salesmen ran when they saw me coming). My life was built around mobility. Everything I owned could fit in a U-Haul. I dreamt of circling the globe in one endless wandering so I wouldn't have to commit to anything or anyone. If I looked myself square in the face, I had to admit that the biggest decision I'd ever made was to buy a used car—and I loved it until the day my mechanic said, "Rust." (I then dumped it faster than you can say, "Howmuchoowanforit?")

How do you expect to make a huge, life-altering decision when you can't decide on little stuff?

More topics to discuss with your shrink . . .

---

42. Alert: Does she like that you can't commit?

One day, you're bound to wonder, *Why does she put up with me? I'm being a total pain in the ass. I can't decide. And although I realize I'm one hell of a catch, there are others who would flip over her and slide a ring on her finger—immediately.*

If you ask her, she'll reply, "There's nobody out there like you" or "Most of the good men are already married or they're gay." But there may be more to it than she knows: She may also be unconsciously playing out her own commitment issues. Perhaps her fears are under the surface, and her way of avoiding them is to find a guy who can't commit. (You.) No matter how many times you break up, she's ready to reconcile. No matter how many fights you initiate, she'll patch it up. You dish it out; she takes it. Why?

First, society makes it easy for her to hide. Everybody's saying, "She's a saint! A martyr! For putting up with you, give her a medal!"

But maybe this is an Uncommitted Woman pattern. As long as she's with a guy who can't commit, she doesn't have to. Maybe she had been attracted to men who turned out to be married, who didn't treat her well, who cheated and lied and hurt her. Perhaps she had moved in with men who promptly (or at least emotionally) moved out. Maybe she rationalized: "Oh, he'll leave his wife." "Everything will change when we live together." "He'll leave his job and move to my city to be with me." "He'll open up once he trusts me in marriage."

You're not the only one with issues. It's time for her to explore her own—and for you to be aware of them. It's counterproductive to imagine that the man is always to blame.

43. *Get your signals straight on monogamy.*

Don't believe in the double standard, as my friend Pam's boyfriend did. "I must know if I can trust you," he said in a determined tone. "You can trust me," she replied lightly. "Even if I'm gone on business," he said, "I must know nothing will happen." "Of course," she replied. "Needless to say, I expect the same from you," she added.

He froze.

"What? But it's different for men," he said. "Different *how?*" she asked. "Men have *needs,*" he began. "Real, physical *urges,*" he said. "Women don't?" she asked. "Let me put it this way," he began, sliding slowly into quicksand. "When I was a boy, my father went to work in the gold mines, deep in the jungle. We kids knew he was fooling around. How could he not, when he was gone four, five months at a time? Ha!" he chortled. (She didn't join in.) "But we would have been astonished if our mother did the same. It would have been wrong. All wrong. Can't you see?"

By the time he said the second "all wrong," the relationship was over.

Another guy described a marriage formula he called "15-10-10-out." It went like this: Commit to one woman for fifteen years of marriage and then get an option for another ten, or move on to another partner for ten and then do the same in ten years. Then marry one more time until death. All this because he hated the notion of sex with one partner until eternity. He mentioned the idea to his girlfriend, who said, "But that's leasing! That's a world made for men! I want marriage!"

So how do you get your signals straight? One married friend said, "I told my then-girlfriend that if I would pledge monogamy, I needed her to commit to keeping our sex life vital. It couldn't feel like she was doing me a favor. I didn't want to hear later on that sex once every ten weeks was her idea of 'a lot of sex.' I didn't want to have to resort to internet porno because we weren't having sex. And I told her that it was one thing not to pursue other women because we were active and another to turn the other way when nothing is happening at home."

Another friend got his signals straight another way. "At one point, my girlfriend and I had a 'What's the Big Fuss About Sex?' talk. We both agreed that it occupied only twenty minutes per week for us—and sometimes not even that—but we were cool with it. For us, our priority was keeping a fun and peaceful home."

The bottom line: Talk about the details, so there's no misunderstanding after you're married.

(More about monogamy later.)

44. No, it's not a jail sentence.

In the middle of all his confused thinking, my friend Todd said, "I recall seeing a man biking in the park with his wife, followed by three kids on their bikes. I don't think he looked particularly unhappy, but I remember thinking, 'Man, that guy is trapped. He's fried. His life's about as exciting as overcooked zucchini.'" I mentioned this to a friend who said, "What the hell are you talking about? The guy on the bike may have been the happiest son of a bitch alive. What makes you think that guy's on death row?"

Another friend: "I used to get really depressed when I'd read a book jacket that said, 'So and so lives with his wife and two children in the Pacific Northwest.' It seemed he'd taken the edge off his life."

Keep your projections in check. Are all married men miserable? Are all single guys happy? Ask yourself, "Just because a man chooses to go through life with a woman, does it mean he's not living an interesting, challenging life?" Ultimately, it's up to you and your lover.

45. Remember that single life was never perfect.

Every rotten date you ever had falls out of your memory the instant your girlfriend wants commitment. All you remember are the transcendent moments: when you and a date steamed up a parked car down by the river or when a woman yanked off her clothes and pulled you into an eerily lit suburban pool at three in the morning.

Take a second to remember how awful dating could be. "I hated the uncertainty of dating," one friend said. "For me, single life was not being tall enough or loud enough. All I remember were trashy parties with superficial people shouting dumb things at one another." "It was an exercise in intimidation," another friend said. For me, it was the letdown of walking into a room, doing the Single Guy Scan (*dzz-ttt, dzzzz-ttt*-ing my eyes around the room for The One) and realizing—once again—that she wasn't there.

Realize that life will never imitate a beer commercial (no matter how hard you want it to). I was hitchhiking on a shoestring vacation to Spain when a carload of blonde Scandinavian women picked me up. "Where you goink?" the driver (in overalls and nothing underneath) asked. "Nowhere in particular," I stammered. "You stay with us, yes?" the driver said. "We have rented house, no. Nothing fancy, yes? Is OK, no?" *Is OK, yes.*

Immediately, my mind was off to the races. How would I decide among the beauties? They were all giggly and bouncy and innocent and eligible. We lit candles, ate dinner, downed a bottle of cheap wine, got ready for bed. Together.

They hopped into bed—in pairs—turned out the lights, said good night, snuggled and kissed and fell asleep. I sat up, scratching my head. *Huh? In a beer commercial, I would have had all five of the women all over me as we cut back to the ball game.*

Beware: The closer you get to commitment, the more you imagine single life really *was* a beer commercial. But it's not, and it wasn't, nor will it ever be. Focus on what you have, not some dumb illusion.

46. *Remember that marriage doesn't have to seem so . . . FINAL.*
Don't do the equivalent of endlessly and aimlessly spinning the car radio dial. You know you're in trouble if you hear a song you like and still can't stop the dial. Then it's just the motion of searching that you find consoling.

Guys struggle to grasp the enormity of the choice. But it's not like the question, "Which CD would I bring if I were to be stranded on a deserted island?" (You guess you'd wing *any* CD Frisbee-style into the great blue beyond.)

Better to think of marrying many women because your wife will, in fact, be many women. First, she's the woman in the tight jeans and pointy-cowboy boots who drives ninety miles-an-hour in her white Bronco. Then she's your bride in the lacy dress. Then she's your lover in the lakeside cabin. Then she's your home girl in the baggy wool sweater. Then she's the woman in labor, shouting obscenities. Then she's the woman nursing your baby. Then she's the woman urging your toddler on as he clops across the floor. Then she's the woman in the hotel room who's still interested in jumping your bones.

Just be sure to take snapshots along the way.

Thinking Marriage

47. *There's no tougher place to be than at someone else's wedding.*

In the midst of my commitment crunch, we were slated to attend my friend Enrico's wedding. We were going to chug around Manhattan on a Circle Line boat, sip champagne, nibble cake, and dance to none other than Dr. John.

I knew trouble was brewing when my girlfriend played out her frustrations over my commitmentphobia on several pairs of shoes before the mirror. "Which ones look better?" she asked. "Uhhmm . . . I like them both?" I said, not able to tell them apart. "Well, I can't stand the whole thing!" she said, changing not only shoes but outfits. Then, just as we were walking out the door, she turned. "I can't take it. I'm not going!" she said. "*They* can get married and they're not half as in love as we are! *Everyone* can get married! Just not *you!* Not *us!* I'm sick of it, and I'm not watching them tie the knot!" "But . . ." I said. "Have fun," she said. "Maybe you'll meet a woman there who you *will* marry."

The weddings we did attend were even more torturous, with everyone saying, "So, you guys are next, huh?" (And God forbid your girlfriend catches the bouquet—a practice many commitmentphobes consider barbaric.) One friend said, "At least half of our breakups came in the wake of weddings. I'd say something like, 'Who's to say they'll be happily married?' or 'Many of those wedding couples are already divorced by now.' "

Those remarks will only spark a fight. Don't go there.

48. Also beware of major holidays.

When the fireworks are blasting and midnight has struck, there's only one thing she wants: a ring. Champagne, Beluga, Godiva . . . forget it. Just grab the nearest cigar band, slip it on her finger, and she's a happy gal.

You can wiggle your way past Christmas, New Year's Eve, and July 4th, but Valentine's Day, it's put up or shut up. "I got engaged the week before Valentine's Day," my friend Kyle said, "because I couldn't handle Sharon's disappointment one more time."

If you're not going to propose on a major holiday (and you know she's anticipating a proposal), you'd better let her know in advance. Deflecting—as though you're a goalie and she's Brett Hull—will not work. Tell her that your relationship shouldn't be governed by dates that pop up on the calendar.

But she knows she'll get "*So?*" calls from her mother or girlfriends. A brutal truth: Another "no-proposal" holiday may be too much for her to take.

49. *Events may precipitate a crisis.*

You're offered a job on the other side of the continent, but there's no way she'll move out there with you in your uncommitted state. She's not about to give up her job and apartment and risk being dumped in a strange city.

Nothing but commitment will work here. "You have to trust that I still love you," said a boyfriend to my friend Pam (before embarking on a new job in a new city). "Meaning?" she asked. "I'm going to go there and be faithful." "And then?" she asked. "And then I'll be back, and we'll be together." "And no promises? No engagement? No proposal?" she asked, incredulous. "Well, no," he said, biting his lip.

She told him to pack his bags and hit the road.

50. *Be alert to "deal breakers."*

Sometimes, while you're wading through your commitment fears, an event throws *The Wrongness of You and Her* into startling light.

Three years into a relationship, my friend Daryl decided to chase his dream of making a short film, so he went back to school part time, wrote a script, and cast and shot the twenty-minute picture. "If we were married," his girlfriend said, "I wouldn't let you do this." *Wham!* It was like a door catching him square in the face. "You'd *what?!* Wouldn't let me make my movie?" That spelled curtains on the relationship.

Or maybe she keeps expecting you to grow up and stop waking up at six on a Saturday morning so you can bike a hundred miles. Or quit camping on a peak so you can see a meteor shower. Or get a real job with real money and real power—when you dropped out of law school because it wasn't your chosen life.

Try this exercise: Name the favorite moments in your life. Now ask her to name hers. If there's no correlation between yours and hers, you may be in trouble. Yours may be eating a cheese sandwich in a hot second-class train spinning through rural Italy. Hers may be eating a four-star room-service meal in a four-star hotel—without an expense account. There's nothing wrong with either vision of a perfect life, but they may not jibe.

Now identify your dream life. Imagine you have enough money for everything from M & Ms to paying off Uncle Sam. How would you fill your day? Would you move? What about your work? Ask her to do the same. Are your dreams similar?

Another good question to ask yourself is, "Am I accepting her for who she is?" (She ought to ask the same question of you.) Maybe you just don't belong together.

EXPECT TO FREAK OUT THE MORNING AFTER YOU BREAK UP WITH HER.

---

51. *If you break up, you may want to come right back.*

You say you need space, and she begrudgingly hands you your freedom. Then *you* flip out. *You* come begging for more. *You* seduce her and wine her and make love to her and obsessively crash at her place every night.

Remember, you are terrified of forever—forever *away* from her is as scary as forever *with* her. You freak. You like having her as your human safety net, so if you free-fall from that high-wire act called dating, you've got a place to land. Breakups are like spikes through your heart. Jealousy: You fear another guy will be all over her the instant you bolt, and maybe he'll be one of those ultra-handsome men, or maybe she'll sleep with him and he'll keep going and going and going—or, worse (much, much worse), he'll be one of those guys in the locker room who refuses to wear a towel because he's so glad to drive every other guy nuts with envy (he even showers facing out so the damned thing wags for everyone to see).

And what about distance? Of all my commitment-related breakups, one stands out. We were in Los Angeles, eating at a Mexican restaurant, when my girlfriend basically said, "Put up or shut up." When I froze, she ran out the door and into our tiny rental car. In a puff of exhaust, she drove back to the hotel without me.

My first reaction was, *Thank God! She's Gone!* But my next reaction was, *Oh, my God! She's Gone!* I dashed outside to Sunset Boulevard. Smog. Billboards and platform shoes everywhere. I returned to our hotel and lunged toward my girlfriend, apologized profusely, and promised to get it together.

FACE WHAT'S WRONG. Say to her, "I will not get back together unless I'm willing _____" (move in together, propose, or whatever). She may say to you, "I will not get back together unless you can_____" (talk out our problems at a couple's therapist, give me a damned ring, and so on).

These are nonnegotiable points for both sides.

---

52. *Don't set up a pattern of fights and resolutions just so you can have the reward: hot sex.*

It's an unhealthy cycle, but all too often couples fall into it. Remember: Sex can muddle your decision.

53. *Loneliness or jealousy may prompt a proposal. But these are not good reasons to get married.*

There's nothing like a lonely night at a bar filled with losers to jolt you to your senses. Drifters are burping in your face while you're stuck to the beer-gooey floor. By the time the peroxide blonde in the pink acrylic sweater and sequined pants sucks the olive from her last martini, you're ready to bolt out the door and back to your girlfriend. You're tempted to blurt out a proposal.

My friend Amy said, "Cliff broke up with me one day after years of badgering him to decide on marriage. Then he bumped into me at a party the next night, and some cute guy was flirting with me, asking me out. The clincher was when Cliff went into the john and found that the other guy had scrawled his love for me in graffiti on the stall wall. The next morning, Cliff was out of control; he left six messages on my machine. By ten-thirty. He proposed two weeks later."

But the engagement was broken before they dashed to the altar.

54. *Expect romantic trickery.*

The year before I proposed, my girlfriend accompanied me to twenty-one baseball games. Considering that she went to only *one* in the first ten years of our marriage, is it fair to say she was engaging in bait and switch?

I loved having her come to games with me, not because she'd argue a call at second, but because her perspective was so different from my own. She commented on which team had the nicest "outfit." She'd talked about the players' thighs and butts. Or she asked deeply philosophical questions about the game, such as why players chew tobacco. And she was there by my side, looking sexy in a baseball cap turned backward, watching the sky turn deep blue then black, listening to the hum of the crowd.

For years, I complained that coming to those games was part of a plot to get me to propose. "Well, yeah," she said. "Just as you're guilty of leading me to believe you'd be my shoe-shopping companion." Touché.

Romantic trickery is part of courtship's playbook—and more of it in marriage will keep the juices flowing.

55. Drown out the voices.

You will feel dizzy from the cyclone of opinions about moving in. Your parents will say to you: "Don't live together! You'll cut off all your options!" Her parents will say to her: "Don't give him everything without a ring!" Your friends will say to you: "Move in! Otherwise, you'll never know how you feel." Her friends will say to her: "Don't move in until he proposes!" She will say to you or you will say to her: "Unless you move in, it's over. I need something more." You'll both say: "I can't even think any more!"

One friend said, "I did a survey. Three out of four people told me not to move in. I was so confused I went away to Vermont to figure things out. I couldn't eat or sleep because I would think one thing one moment and another thing the next." Finally, he realized he had to move in, or he'd lose the relationship—and his sanity.

56. *Have you moved in without knowing it?*

After a short while, my girlfriend and I were spending every night together. After work, I'd exercise, shower, grab a suit for the next day, and bike to her place. We'd eat dinner, read, and make love. (Less often, she'd come to my place—a studio with a lot of character and a bathroom that she considered suitable only for an excon.) To me, this routine was heaven.

But eventually, every "hello" carried a subtext of an unspoken ultimatum: *Either we move in together or we end the relationship.* I stalled and hemmed and hawed. I kept pointing out to her how impossibly high New York rents were. Basically, I was terrified of cutting off my options—and hearing my parents and friends rip into me on the phone. One day, she called me from a block away to say that she'd found the perfect pad for us to live in together. More space. A working fireplace. High ceilings. A manageable rent when chopped in two. An Italian landlord (she knew my soft spot for anything Italian).

Reluctantly, I went to look at it. After twenty minutes, the real estate broker started tapping her watch. I paced back and forth and took a deep breath, walked into the bedroom, and signaled to my girlfriend. "It'll be so romantic," she said. I sighed. "You'll love living with me," she said. I exhaled. "I won't bark at you to take out the garbage," she said. "I'm keeping my place," I qualified. She nodded. "I'm not giving it up," I added. She threw her arms around me—but I was numb. "So . . . yes?"

I felt like I'd just dived from a fifty-foot cliff into an unknown sea.

We walked around the apartment. No, this wasn't how I'd pictured it. *Why hadn't I found the pad? Why couldn't I take the initiative?* But I was slowly learning that reality was one hell of a lot sloppier than the glossy perfection of my imagination. Besides, I felt a stirring in my chest. We'd taken a step—no matter how we had gotten there, we'd arrived.

We sat on the bare floor, and I drummed my fingers. "You want me to run out for pizza and beer?" I asked. She wrapped her arm over my shoulder and said, "It's gonna be all right." "I know," I said, without conviction. "Lemme get us some pizza and beer." Then she ruffled my hair and laughed at my male stupidity. I began to feel OK. Even a bit better than OK.

57. Beware of saying, "Well, just for a while."

Her lease is expiring so you say, "Live with me—just until you find another place." No sooner said than done.

For the ensuing weeks, she halfheartedly scours the newspaper for another apartment while you two have morning coffee. "These rents are sick," she says whenever you glance at her. You study a box score. "Sick," she says. You read a movie review. "Sick." "OK, OK. So, stay a while longer," you say.

Yeah, living together is working out and you're saving money and getting closer (to each other, to commitment), but you're in the danger zone: You didn't make the decision. Careful now, or this could haunt you later on.

You never want to feel an imaginary fish hook in your mouth.

•   •   •

58. Don't let your mind race you into trouble.

When you first shut the door of your shared apartment, you notice a deep, profound silence.

"You OK?" she says. "I'm OK," you say. She knows you're not OK and takes you by the hand, leads you to the mattress, and makes wild, passionate love to you.

This is good. This is very good. Your brain stops quivering like a bowl of Jell-O on a subway.

And then you notice something nice. She smiles differently. This is what she's wanted. Commitment from you.

Gulp. You ask yourself, *What will she want next?*

A baby. Somewhere between what a woman says and what a man hears, the words change to "Let's get married *and have a baby.*" You've been in your new digs nineteen seconds, and you're already worried about a baby wrecking it. You think she intends to destroy what you've just created: *A life built around adventure and sex.*

Nobody's bothered to tell you: Fatherhood is no reason not to get married. In fact, it's a great reason *to* get married. The day you're teaching your kid to pitch a baseball is the day it all comes into focus for a lot of guys.

59. Don't keep one foot out the door.

Say you keep your former apartment (as I did). She knows it's your escape hatch. When things get tough, you bolt. If you fight, you're outta there. When you say you're going for a walk, she thinks you're walking to your place to call another woman or to hash it over with a buddy. One woman told me, "I could tell how well we were doing by the amount of clothes he kept in 'our' apartment. If his closet was full, I knew he was serious. When the closet emptied, his interest had waned. It pissed me off."

But maybe you live in a tight real estate market; if you two break up and she has the lease, you're homeless. (Giving up your apartment in a tight urban real estate market is akin to letting go of an igloo on a subzero polar night.) How do you show her your belief without moving in all the way? You assign a new role for your old apartment. Use it as an office for work. Leave your electric guitar and an amp and nothing else. Take all your clothes out—and don't let them migrate back in. Differentiate roles, so she can clearly see your commitment to her.

60. Know your response to, "Well, are you two living together?"

Maybe you didn't get a new pad together—so it's not obvious that you're sharing a place. Well, after your stuff has migrated into her apartment or hers into yours, people *will* take note. Friends will spot your suits in her closet or her bras poking out of your dresser (and, yes, they'll check to see if her tampons and birth control pills are in your medicine cabinet). In a sly voice, they'll ask about your living arrangements.

Coordinate your responses. When my friends Michelle and Jack were asked this question at a dinner party, she blurted, "Yes!" while he choked, "No."

The result was ugly. Dead silence. Michelle blanched. Jack got up and took some plates to the kitchen, and, naturally, the friends asked Michelle, "What's wrong with this creep? He doesn't know if you're living together?" She said, "Well, I'm not so sure we are anymore!"

61. *She may be the one who panics.*

With everyone screaming at her, "Yo, girl! You've given him everything! He's got to put up or shut up!" she may not realize that for the guy, living together is a step toward marriage.

She calms down. Then she's hears of a woman who lived with a man for seventeen years (he was known throughout his borough as "Mr. Rental"), and she freaks again. Or she panics that it's all "Make Believe Forever." My friend Lisa said, "I helped Nick renovate his loft. When we were replastering his walls, he said, 'Let's plant a time capsule.' *Very* romantic idea. As we closed up the wall, Nick said, 'Someone will find this bottle in a hundred years.'

"Not fair! I flipped out! He was waving a hundred years before my eyes! I was picturing us married, having kids, grandchildren . . . and we still weren't engaged!"

62. **With living together comes familiarity, and with familiarity comes stuff like farting.**

The time will come when your woman realizes you are, indeed, a living, breathing, farting creature—not a piece of Greek statuary.

On our first weekend away together, we visited my girlfriend's brother, who served us a dinner of chili, rice and beans, and red bean ice cream for dessert (was this a conspiracy?).

The result was predictable: My girlfriend and I were about to burst, but neither of us would admit we had intestines. "Hey," I said, getting up from the table after dessert, "I'm going to check out the stars." I went outside and let loose and then came back in. A moment later, my girlfriend said, "I think I left the TV on in the living room." Me (five minutes later): "I have to check my messages.

Back in a flash." Her: "Did I ever show you my New Mexican silver belt? Let me get it." By the time we were in bed, we'd exhausted every plausible excuse to bolt out of the room—but that didn't stop us from trying. "I love the sound of crickets. See you in a second."

Much later, after you've sworn your life and love to this woman, the problem will be *too much* familiarity. You'll learn to ignore improprieties and create little windows of romance so you can keep your love fresh.

63. *Pay no attention to the brutal statistics.*

Somebody is bound to thump you on the head with a survey: Couples who cohabitate before marriage do worse than couples who don't live together first.

But marriage is about nothing if not optimism. It's healthy to think, *I'm going to beat the odds.* (Just weeks before getting married, a guy I know said, "I'm taking it day to day. Best not to think too long term." He was divorced three years later.)

There are advantages to living together. My friend Ricky, who's an extreme skier, said, "Before I do anything extreme, I climb up from the bottom and take a look. I see all the obstacles and know where I can take the forty-foot jump and where I can't." Translate that into marriage, and you've got my feelings about living together.

Besides, the alternative doesn't seem so perfect. "You hear about these people who don't live together," my friend Daryl said. "There's the hubbub of engagement, followed by the hysteria of planning the wedding, followed by the bliss of the honeymoon, and then they get back and *kerplunk!* They're roommates!"

Here are a few tips for living together. Let it all hang out. Don't treat it like a test, or you'll choke and not be yourself. Can you two create a space in which you're both comfortable? Can you mesh her vision with your own? Go shopping. How does it feel to make small decisions together? Now jump in with both feet and buy something together that can't be divided—a couch, a dining table—but not something lightweight like a popcorn maker. If it's her place, don't be afraid to make it yours too. For her, it's like playing house as a little girl. Help her move all the furniture around until 2 A.M.—a woman's fantasy.

64. Some women won't move in without a ring.

"I couldn't take a step back," one woman said. "I felt he had to offer me everything up front." "Men need to chase," said another. "Only dumb women move in. Give a man the path of least resistance, and he'll take it," said a third.

Granted, these remarks may drive you nuts (and you may not go for it—I wouldn't have). On the other hand, my friend Warren said, "Gina's unwillingness to live together first is part of her charm. It's what makes her a special package. I can deal with it."

DON'T PLAY THE PERCENTAGE GAME. My friend Harry kept asking, "You can't get 100 percent of what you want in one woman. What do you get: 75 percent, 80 percent, 85 percent, 90 percent?"

He wasn't ready for marriage. (The woman you marry is not a commodity.)

---

65. Is her mother grilling you?

The subtext of everything she'll say is, *Don't waste one more nanosecond of my precious daughter's eligible years.* The subtext of everything you say is, *Who the hell are you to tell me what to do with my life?* All this makes for tangy exchanges that (hopefully) won't get out of hand.

Don't bend too far to please your future mother-in-law or you'll lose yourself, resent it later, and take it out on your girlfriend. Stand your ground. Explain that you love her daughter and will work things out, but don't let her pry into your personal matters.

But before you get all high and mighty about her intrusiveness, squint into the future. Imagine how tough it would be to watch *your* daughter in a similar situation.

66. Don't let her side with your mother

She thinks that your mother can pound some sense into you. So, she drops a hint here or there about what a Neanderthal you are (your mother agrees). Soon, the two women are conspiring in hour-long phone conversations behind your back, plotting how to shake you to your senses.

You call your mother and say, "Steer clear, Mom," and she replies, "Well, if you had proposed by now, I wouldn't have to be in the picture!" You: "It's my life." Her: "Fine. Good. She's a saint. You're a schmutz. You don't deserve her anyway." (When you tell your girlfriend what your mother says, she just smiles.)

Set some clear limits. She can speak with your mother but not conspire behind your back. You need similar rules later on, when you're married—or it will be fair game for your mother to say to her, "How do you put up with him?"

---

6 THINGS HER MOTHER MAY SAY (BETWEEN BITES OF THANKSGIVING MASHED POTATOES)

1. "Not everyone waits for lightening to strike before they get married!"
2. "My wedding dress is in the attic. Collecting dust. Decomposing. Fading."
3. "Her father and I may be dead soon."
4. "Of all my friends, I'm the only one not to have grandchildren."
5. "I just decided I'm going to give her baby toys to charity, so someone who *is* married and who *wants to have children* can use them."
6. "I should only live to see it!"

---

67. You will have exceedingly difficult moments.

Nothing unhinged me more than when my girlfriend brought me to the hospital to visit her uncle, who was dying of cancer. Everyone described him as one of those rare creatures who touched everyone with his kindness, and I wanted to meet him—but not under those circumstances. His hospital room was littered with bleeping monitors and IV drips and flowers and cards. My girlfriend's eyes welled as she hugged him, and he propped himself on a pillow to speak. We visited for a while until the nurses suggested that we leave. And then her uncle said, "I'd like to have a minute alone with you." I prayed he was talking to someone else, but he nodded at me again.

He told me he knew he was dying and now was not the time for pretending. But he had to know, man to man, if I was going to marry his niece. He asked me to take his hand and give him my word.

I shifted on my feet. I took a deep breath and wondered how to reply. I realized that no one has the luxury of infinite time. I couldn't just wait for the decision to hit me without expecting consequences. My *indecision* was like dropping an M-80 into a pond: The ripple effect had reached relatives and friends. I also realized that her family might one day be my own—and I wondered if I'd ever be forgiven. No, I wasn't living in a vacuum.

Finally, I told him that I was sure I would marry her, but I didn't know when. Clearly, this was not the response he'd wished for, but he shook my hand softly.

68. Is your own clock ticking, too?

Much is made of her biological clock—and rightly so. But it's easy to forget that men also have an internal clock. No, not necessarily to have a baby (although you'd like to be able to bend over for your *kid's* kid without toppling over). You may feel an urgency to find an ideal mate, too—only nobody seems to notice.

If you wait too long, there'll be a moment when people stop

looking at you as a single guy and think of you as a bachelor. You want to be on the near side of that line. Growing up, everybody had an "Uncle Harry" who was an eternal bachelor. You don't want to become an Uncle Harry. Professionally single.

69. Code red! Code red! She's turning thirty!

In case you're not familiar with the rules of this planet, thirty is a huge milestone for a woman. My friend Steve said, "I was living with a woman who turned thirty. I came home, and it was as if an ax was hanging over my head. There was no avoiding it. We started to fight constantly."

When she turns thirty, there may be only one word: *baby*. It will freak you out. My friend Carl said, "When Jeanne was twenty-eight, I mentioned babies, and she said, 'Isn't a cat enough?' Suddenly, she turned thirty and had me checking out little blue-and-green checkered sweaters in baby stores. 'Maybe we ought to buy this. Just so we have it for when the time is right.' I was stupefied." One day, you're reading the paper when you come across an article on fertility after thirty, thirty-five, forty, and you gulp real hard. *What if you don't marry her? Then you may have messed up her life!*

You can tell her she doesn't look or act thirty, and she'll say, "But *I am* thirty." There's no way around this one. It's not just that she'll point to a vein under her eye or a tiny bit of extra flesh above her elbow or knee. (You haven't noticed any of these signs; now you feel guilty—as if you caused them.)

But the bonuses of an over-thirty-year-old woman are plenty. Women ripen. There's a resonance that may not have been there before. And your thirty-year-old girlfriend may really be into sex in a way she wasn't in her twenties. A light goes off in your head. Sex Ed. Older woman; hot sex drive.

70. Don't tease her with "a ring" before "the ring."

It's a stall tactic. You want to ease the pressure so you promise to buy her a ring that says, *Someday soon, we'll get the real thing — but it's not an engagement ring, and it's not a wedding band, and it's not an eternity ring.*

Don't do it.

71. Be careful not to push her buttons inadvertently.

You're shopping for hammocks in a Mexican market when the craftsman says, "Which size do you want? Solo? *Matrimonio?*" You say, "Definitely *matrimonio.*"

Whoa! Her eyes start spinning like one-armed bandits that just hit the jackpot. So you dash her off to the nearest bar, saying, "We've got to catch the World Cup! It's Italy versus Holland! The whole world's watching!" And she's still mumbling, *"Matrimonio."*

You will sometimes feel the world is conspiring against you, pushing you into that wild, foreign land, *Matrimonio.* (You're right; the world is trying to push you.)

72. Figure out ways of dealing with your claustrophobia.

When your palms sweat, your stomach tightens, or your eyes dilate because life is getting too cozy, you think, *If only I could helicopter ski in the Canadian Rockies.*

Try intermediary measures. Take a subway ride to a remote

neighborhood. Drive fifteen minutes to somewhere you've never been. Sometimes a quick hit of freedom does the trick.

73. Test what you feel is the relationship's weakness.

One of my biggest fears was traveling with my girlfriend for the rest of my life. My idea of travel was to land in a country I knew nothing about with only a day pack and a guidebook. Hers was to go to a beach, lay in a lounge chair under an umbrella, order drinks and lunch, and read the day away.

I wasn't sure if this was a deal-breaker, so I decided to test it. I outfitted my girlfriend with a backpack and hiking boots and arranged for us to trace part of the ancient caravan route across the Turkish desert. This was one of my long-time dreams. We stopped in a remote village of mud huts. We were invited to stay in a home with striped textiles on the floor, walls, and ceiling; a toothless grandmother at the loom in one corner; and the evening's dinner clucking near the front door. Our host brought out a yogurt drink so thick you could turn the cup upside down and nothing would fall out. "My house is your house. Stay with us. Be our guests," he said. "This is heaven," I said to my girlfriend. "Let's stay for a week or two." She whispered into my ear, "Either we sleep in the car, or this relationship will end the instant you get me out of this goddamned desert."

That night, when we stewed in the front seat of our rented car, my girlfriend said, "Get it through your head: You can't just drag me to Timbuktu or wherever the hell we are and expect me to enjoy it." I realized then (or maybe it was when we hit a hotel that wouldn't have received a star even in *The Primitive Hotel Lovers'*

Guide to the Universe) that it isn't necessary for the woman you love to be absolutely *everything*. I was searching for an exotic beauty who could bob up in an ocean, pull back her wet hair and say something dirty in Italian, discuss Tolstoy *and* the NBA play-offs, a woman who could hike up K-2 with a passed-out Sherpa lashed to her back. But in marriage, you don't *want* one person to do everything. You'll have friends who pick up where your wife leaves off.

What traits are vital in your mate? Her sense of loyalty, honesty, and responsibility? Her ability to turn you on and be turned on by you? Her determination to make it through tough patches? Think it through.

OK, so I'll never raft down the Amazon with my wife. But we've worked out compromises. When we go for a beach vacation, I throw on my hiking boots and four-wheel to the nearest rain forest for a day while she parks herself in a beach chair and doesn't move.

74. Act out your fantasies with your girlfriend now.

My friend Eric told me he had been obsessed by the proverbial Do-*it*-in-an-Airplane-Lavatory Fantasy. Sex at thirty thousand feet. Passengers not knowing. A flight attendant knocking on the door. The threat of someone finding out.

As his relationship with Julia went into its second, and then third year, he realized that there might *never* be a chance before marriage to fulfill his fantasy with a nameless beauty who had squiggled into the seat beside him. He decided to live it out.

On an overnight flight to Europe, he whispered to his girlfriend, "Let's do it in the john." "Everyone will know," she protested. "No, they won't," he said raspily. "You go first. I'll wait one minute. I'll rap on the door: Tap, tap-tap, tap. You'll let me in. Then you'll leave first and I'll leave a few minutes later."

The bathroom was cramped, the light was unflattering, it smelled like airplane lavatory, and he accidentally flushed the toilet with his knee and the *whoosh* was about as erotic as triggering a car alarm. So what? It was fantasy brought to life. When they were back in their seats, Eric said, "We did it! I've always wanted to do that—and it was amazing!" (Within days, he claimed he'd found the cure for jet lag, to which Julia merely rolled her eyes.)

Unrealized fantasies can hold a man back from sharing his life with one woman. Live out the harmless ones now—*and* later, during marriage. Kiss and grope in department store changing rooms or under the bleachers at minor league baseball games. Keep it hot. You get the picture.

75. You or she should never decide under an ultimatum.

Warning: Neurotic Land. Stay away.

The first ultimatum was the most frightening for me because it turned out to be movable. I tried to decide, couldn't, and decided I couldn't decide—and she immediately moved back the ultimatum to a later date. (If there's anything worse than an ultimatum, it's a series of *sliding ultimatums* which only prolong the agony.)

Finally, I grew so sick of ultimatums (and of hurting her through my indecision) that I broke up just so I wouldn't be delivered one again. I flew to visit my brother, who was then a graduate student at Berkeley. At the inn where I was staying, the dark-haired receptionist, a beauty made more mysterious by her reading glasses and a tome on some obscure philosopher, got my attention. She was studiously sexy. We talked for hours. Pheromones shot back and forth between us. Ironically, her boyfriend had given her an ultimatum, and *she* couldn't decide either.

We said goodnight and decided we'd meet the next morning for coffee at her reception desk. We seemed to have a lot in common: our hatred of ultimatums. Our fatigue with breakups. Our desire to rip each other's clothes off. The next morning, we flirted and laughed and both guessed this might turn into something. Suddenly, the hotel phone rang. "Call for you," she said gloomily, handing me the phone. It was my girlfriend, hoping to hop a plane for San Francisco in three hours. "Please don't come out here. I can't hurt you any more. I can't stand the pressure. I'm tired of not deciding," I said. "OK," she said. "That was the last ultimatum. Can I come out? Please, I promise, no more." Sure.

Without an ultimatum hanging over my head, I could breathe again, and we drove to Napa Valley. Amid the hills tumbling with vineyards, I realized I had hoped to evade the pressure and the sense of being trapped. Feeling more unencumbered, I proposed a month later.

Sure, I've heard of men who needed a sharp nudge in the ribs—and they're still married. But there are some of us (and I'm one) who need to make decisions on our own.

•   •   •

IT'S GOT TO BE YOUR DECISION. No, you're not deciding to make her happy, her mother happy, your mother happy, or anybody's mother happy. If the decision isn't to make you happy, the shit will hit the fan. Big Time.

---

76. Does she play mind games with you to finagle a proposal?

The day will come when your girlfriend says, "I've had it! I'm out of here! Good-bye! I'm going to Puerto Rico with Janice. And don't even think of leaving a message on my machine while I'm gone!"

This gets under your skin big time—especially if Janice is a dude magnet who's only beach garment is a thong that could fit into a cigarette box. You envision the worst: the two women shielding their eyes in their lounge chairs as they flirt with tanned guys with Speedos and washboard abs.

It may bother you considerably less if your girlfriend does as mine did and heads off to Death Valley with her brother (her brother)! That trip failed to rev nightmares from the hinterlands of my mind (I envisioned endless drives through salt flats and gas stations attended by lizard-skinned geezers staring off into nowhere). What *did* get me was when she hired a chisel-faced, former Telluride ski instructor/model to paint her work studio. Brainwashed from porno, I knew the House Painter Always Gets the Girl (so does the plumber, the electrician, the cop, and the pizza delivery man—often all at once). She didn't let on that he was actually gay.

Romantic games work. Jealousy (in moderation) is for her like throwing an off-speed pitch in between a slew of blazing fast balls.

77. *Ask yourself, Does she love me for the right reasons?*

Ask her, "Why do you love me?" When I asked my girlfriend, I realized that she loved me for who I would become as much as who I was. She wanted me to get on with expressing myself. Living—not warming up for life. I loved her vision of my future. It's one of the reasons I married her. I realized she would always challenge me to take risks I might not ordinarily take.

Now it's your turn. Take a minute to think about what it is you really love about her. Then tell her. I said to my girlfriend, "I love your girlishness, that you haven't been wrecked by the world. I love your bizarre cynicism that's not bitter and almost sweet. I love your laugh and how you see the shadows, not just the objects. But I don't love that when we talk about marriage, you become pushy, almost uncaring of my perspective (and ridiculing of it). You shut off and become distant. It's almost like you become another person."

Though this may seem like an obvious exercise to you, it's not. Maybe the qualities you love about her aren't those she values (oops, then you're in trouble). But maybe what you love about her is what she loves most about herself. Perhaps the person she has become during this Marry-Me-Now-Now-NOW! phase isn't who she hopes to be, either. Sometimes you (as a couple) have veered off course while getting to commitment; this understanding will bring you back on target.

78. *She may tempt you by saying you can have flings as a married man. Don't believe her.*

One buddy said that his girlfriend promised he could have a few discreet affairs once they were married. "Here are the conditions," she said. "It'll be like a European marriage. Don't fall in love. Don't let me know. Don't embarrass me. End it after a night or two." He had just one question: "I assume you want reciprocal rights?" "No," she said, "that's not what I'm after."

Lust without love sounded like a pretty good deal to him and, bang-bang, he was engaged and married.

For a few years, he had no inclination to take her up on the offer. But after eight years of marriage, the thought intrigued him.

He mentioned this to his wife before a business trip. She said, "If you ever screw another woman, I'm out the door. That was then, this is now." "But . . ." he said. "Tell me if this sounds fair," she said. "I've got the baby at the pediatrician while you're in Dallas getting done by Debbie in the back boardroom." When he said, "Those were our terms!" she said, "OK, go ahead if you think it's important to you. But if you want to play around, I'm going to also." "Ah . . . forget it," he said.

DON'T LET YOUR BED TURN INTO CAMP DAVID. Some women treat the lull after sex as Negotiation Time. She may say, "So, are you any closer to deciding?" (You may have been until she said that.)

You're going to have to establish No Negotiation Times, too, or your relationship will disintegrate. (Granted, making love triggers her "What next?" reflex. But it is also the Snooze Reflex in most men.)

Now establish Negotiation Times. Pick a special time, say, a dinner out. "Sometimes I want a walk in the park to be a walk in

*the park," one buddy said. "Or lying in bed to be lying in bed. I
don't want other stuff to seep in. I'll say, 'I want to hear what you
have to say. Let's go out for dinner. Write a list if you'd like so we
can hit all your concerns.' Then I'll be psychically prepared. It's
like my knowing a week in advance I'll have to work late instead
of finding out at 6 P.M."*

79. Settle your religious differences now.

My friend Bev said, "I made it very clear to Dan that I was a
Christian before we got serious at all. I said, 'If you have a problem
with that, then I don't even want to go further. I want my kids to
share my religion.' He said, 'Fine with me. I don't feel strongly
either way.'"

And then there's the "both religions" option. My friend Nina
said, "Nathan and I brought up our kids with love and respect for
both families' religions. One of use would have felt cheated, otherwise."

Enter: your parents and hers. "We waited too long to talk it
over," said my friend Ted. "My uncle, a deacon who's Angelican
by conversion, was slated to marry us. But Phoebe wouldn't go for
the prewedding religious training, and before long, everyone was
in a huff and my mother was saying we were evil and were living
in sin, and my father was saying we'd burn in hell. Now, fifteen
years later, they think we're great together."

It can get really ugly. When my friend Greg brought his future
wife home, his father took him outside and told him, "If you
marry her, we will consider you dead. We have our religion, and

she has hers. Better that you were to marry a heroin addict! Or even a whore! We will cut off all relations—and I don't even want you at my funeral." (Tough to enforce that one.)

Greg and his girlfriend got engaged and then married (without his parents' presence), but a seed had been planted. When they had babies, everyone suffered. But it wasn't until years later, when he heard his father was dying, that he and his parents finally got back together.

What an impossible situation—but not unusual. Early on (way before you get to the rings) is the time for you and the woman you love to be brutally honesty about your religious needs.

80. Prenuptials can end your relationship before you're married.

My friend Deana had been going through her boyfriend's endless marital deliberations when he one day said, "I'm just afraid of losing everything. If you're up to signing a prenup, then I'm game." It wasn't romantic, and it wasn't quite a proposal, but she said, "Let's do it." ("I *caved*," she said later.)

A few weeks later, she held in her trembling hands a document that seemed to her about as readable as the Declaration of Independence spelled backward in Swahili. She gave it to two lawyers, one of whom said, "This doesn't pass the stomach test." ("Meaning?" she asked. "It makes me feel queasy," he replied.) The other said, "You can sign. But if you do, you must also sign a disclaimer stating that I advised you against it."

Huh. Not so friendly .

My friend Louanne had a similar experience. "I knew he

came into the relationship with the loft and the earnings and the cars and the house in the country, so I said, 'OK, I'll take a look at a prenup.' But I never expected it to get so harrowing. We left the lawyer's office together and walked out onto the street. I was dizzy, shaking. Then I turned to the man I loved, tears streaming down my face: 'I feel like we've tied the knot, had a kid, it's over, you hate me, I hate you, and I'm out in the world, trying to find an apartment in New Jersey.'" Eventually, they hammered out a workable agreement. "Our lawyer said, 'Let's handle the fears. Let's put in automatic joint custody of a child should you have one. This is all a warm-up for the things you'll negotiate in marriage.'

"We discovered that any little thing that's been pushed under the carpet will come up when your biggest financial buttons are being pressed. Maybe it's better to know your divorce design beforehand."

And what if the situation is reversed (she's got the dough, and you've got *nada*). My pal Eric said, "I knew going into the marriage that she had a million times more in assets than me. But all of a sudden, we were sitting at her family lawyer's office. The lawyer said, 'I know you two are happy now. But lots of couples start out happy! Hell, we all do!' He then held up his ringless hand. 'But divorce is a fact. It's important that someone protect what's his—or, in this case, hers. How do you know,' he said, his gaze going toward my fiancée, 'that he won't tromp off with another woman the week after you tie the knot? It happens, you know.'

"My fiancée pulled me aside and said, 'You all right?' I whispered, 'I know you've got more than I do. But that's not why I'm marrying you. I'm sorry, but I refuse to go into marriage acknowledging that divorce is a possibility. That's the way I am. I'm not going to leave you—ever. We're going to grow old together. And if you don't believe me, find another guy.'" (They got married without a prenup and, sixteen years later, have three kids—and two separate bank accounts because he doesn't want their money to mix.)

Here are a few considerations if you or she wants a prenup. Hire your own lawyers so neither of you will feel betrayed or favored. Never sign while under emotional turmoil or the agreement may not hold up later on. Remember that the agreement can be modified as the marriage changes; it's not written in stone. Most of all, tread very, *very* lightly. You could blow the whole relationship and not need a prenup because there won't be a marriage to protect.

IS MOM RIGHT? *One hesitant guy asked his mother what she thought of his girlfriend. She put it in plain English: "Take away the sex and you could see straight. You wouldn't be with her."*

---

81. Stop pretending to be someone you aren't.
You don't want her to believe that you'll always cancel business meetings so you can accompany her to a White Sale.

My friend Sally said, "He put me and our relationship up on a pedestal while we dated and lived together, then kicked it out but good the day we married. I couldn't believe it. He hated my cooking. He hated my cleaning. He criticized my every action. I said, 'Why'd you fool me before?! I wish you'd just been yourself and saved me the trouble!'"

82. If it's truly holding you back, reveal your deep, dark secret.

Sometimes a man will think, I can't get married without coming clean. It doesn't seem honest. If that's the case, throw the ball into her court and let her decide if she can live with your past error.

One friend simply couldn't pop the question before he told his girlfriend of an affair he had with a man. It took a few weeks for her to acclimate, and some frank discussions, they've been very happily married for ten years and have a baby.

83. Don't hold her hostage to her past.

One friend admitted that he'd grilled his girlfriend about her ex-lovers until she could take it no more. "You really want to know?!" He nodded. "You're not going to hold it against me?" He nodded. "Well, OK." Then she told him of cheating on past boyfriends, trysts with married men, an affair with an executive on his paper-strewn desk, a relationship with her bisexual hairdresser (he died of AIDS; she tested negative) and having oral sex with well-endowed anonymous man in a stall in a nightclub bathroom. He wished he hadn't known any of it (especially the nightclub encounter); he even considered revenge (he hadn't been nearly as promiscuous); but with time, he realized that people can change—and he had to accept her for who she is, not who she had been. Now, years later, they're a solid couple.

Part of trust is trusting what to say and what not to say. You have to think, *Whatever led her to this point, those are the experiences that made her who she is.*

P.S. Never ask if you don't want to know—and you definitely don't want to know some things. That means, No vivid descriptions of Penises from Her Past (in fact, no nonvivid descriptions, either).

P.P.S. Don't ever give her your "number" or ask her for hers. (Your "numbers" are how many lovers you've had in the past.)

IF SHE ASKS HOW SEX WAS WITH A PAST GIRLFRIEND, YOUR REPLY SHOULD BE: "NOTHING GREAT. NOT LIKE US." OR "I CAN'T EVEN REMEMBER."

---

84. Ask yourself if you're holding back because of a past relationship.

My friend Eric was in Could-Not-Decide mode with his girlfriend when he realized his past might be holding him back. Five years before, he'd broken up with his college girlfriend, Francesca—and it ended ugly. Francesca called him night and day, hysterical, sometimes drunk or drugged, threatening suicide if they didn't get back together. He felt caught. They'd make up and get back together and two hours later he'd think, *This is wrong. This is not what I want.*

But when Francesca attempted suicide, something snapped in Eric, too. "For a long time, I was afraid to get involved with any woman. After a few months, I'd break it off. I never told anyone what had happened. I felt guilty. I had promised her a life together—and I'd failed to live up to it.

"I realized I was terrified of bad endings in general (the 'worse' part of 'for better or worse'), that I was lured toward beginnings (when your stomach is churning over whether she will go on a date with you). I was addicted to *wondering* as opposed to *knowing*."

Sure, Eric's past is dramatic, but life happens—nobody is exempt, and your past relationships may *feel* as dramatic to you. Getting to marriage is like anything else: It's gonna take some effort. You've got to cut those ropes that are tethering you.

85. You may have a Ms. Rebound in your life.

When you come closer to making a complete commitment, you may start to view a past girlfriend with great nostalgia. And horniness. And an unreal, glossy, glowing image of what had been.

So you may let your fingers do the dialing. You can't believe yourself as you say, "Hey, how's it goin'?", and then feel that same rush of emotion you felt months or years past.

My friend Chris had a Ms. Rebound. They were together for two years in college, and then she left him for his roommate's brother whom she subsequently married (ouch). Chris tried unsuccessfully to delete her from his memory bank. When she got separated, then divorced, she swung back into his life. She begged for forgiveness. She swore she would never leave him again. But now that she was available (and since Chris wasn't entirely ready for marriage), he didn't get involved with her again. However, in the thick of a committed relationship, he obsessively thought, *Why didn't I give her another chance?*

Yeah, the grass is greener and the beer is better in Bavaria. But the thing to ask yourself is this, "Although I'm drawn to her, why should it end any differently?" Unless you've changed or she's changed, forget it!

86. If it's that bad, get your ass into therapy.

I was desperate. I called a friend and asked if he could recommend a therapist. Two days later, I found myself glancing both ways before ringing the bell of a basement office in a New York brownstone. A small, Germanic man with oversized glasses and a baggy cardigan sweater ushered me in. There was a desk, a couch, and two Lazy-Boy lounge-type chairs facing one another. And a box of tissues near one of the chairs (mine) and an aquarium tank filled with crickets in the corner—as if he was daring me to waste time by asking why he had crickets for pets. He glanced at me as if to say, *So . . .*

"I can't decide whether or not to get married," I blurted. "I've been this way a while—well, too long—and I'm driving everyone nuts. And I just can't decide."

He nodded, but didn't say anything. I whipped through a rapid synopsis of my vacillations, the problem of our different religions, how everyone viewed me as Mr. Commitmentphobe, and all the while, he looked, well, bored. At the end of my long-winded soliloquy, he said, "And where are you from?" "Why do you ask?" I said. "How about your parents, your siblings." I started to gloss over my past, but he simply wouldn't have it. He smiled kindly and said, "You're under way too much pressure. But it's going to take some time to unravel this. I prohibit you from proposing while you're under this duress." I tried to hold back from smiling but couldn't. "Really? You mean, doctor's orders?" I asked. He smiled warmly. "She may be the one, but she may not be," he said. "Let's discover together. See what we see."

The bottom line: You've got to know yourself before you can dream of tying the knot. And knowing yourself involves scraping off all your romantic illusions and finding the equivalent of bare wood underneath. Until then, you're searching for the perfection in her that will make you whole—and that's why you keep going round in circles.

87. But don't get mired in psychobabble.

The entire "My Shrink Says . . ." game can get you into trouble. You: "My shrink says you suffocate me because you've got unresolved abandonment conflicts. He says you pull everyone you love too close!" She: "Well, mine says your anger stems from frustration that your parents won't pick up the phone and say, 'I love you!'" You: "Mine says you were promiscuous in retaliation for your father's womanizing!" She: "Mine says you were too sheltered and should have sowed your wild oats but you were afraid of your mother's rejection!"

Pretty soon, your bed turns into the Battle of the Shrinks. "And in this corner, weighing in at one hundred, seventy-five dollars per hour . . ."

Keep your shrinks to yourself.

88. Don't mentally undress another woman in front of the woman you love.

You're walking past a beautiful woman who's not wearing a bra under her T-shirt. You suddenly realize, *I will never fondle breasts other than my wife's for the rest of my life.* (As the song goes, "Not for just an hour. Not for just a day. Not for just a year. But Al-ways . . .") Or, a sexy flight attendant leans over and asks, "Is there anything else I can get you?"

When you're not with the woman you love, you can mentally undress another woman all you want. When she's around, control yourself. Her radar is on high frequency when it comes to this stuff. Would you like it if you caught her eyes fixed on some guy's crotch? I know: if your weenie is bigger, you couldn't care less. . . .

89. It's OK to do nutty stuff. It gets you ready for real commitment.

For our first Valentine's Day, I gave my girlfriend snowshoes that I'd lashed together to form a heart and a pair of bright pink boxer shorts that were big enough for a sumo wrestler (setting some sort of record in ridiculousness). She cooed, "Ohh . . . How sweet. Snowshoes. And these shorts, they may fit."

Thank God for all those quirky chemicals purring through your veins because of excessive sex. Neither of us considered that she, being a southern girl, considered fifty-nine degrees a cold front and trudging through snow, torture. Neither of us wondered why I'd gotten boxers (she put them on; I tugged them off).

Later on, you'll get practical and wish you weren't.

90. *Make two lists.*

I called my dad. I told him I was getting close to proposing. I told him that the mood had hit me when I was throwing fly balls to my girlfriend while she was wearing the Valentines boxer shorts, a T-shirt, and a baseball cap. My dad seemed unimpressed, especially when I hurriedly told him of another instance when I felt the urge: She had rolled down the car window near a farm we were passing and said, "I just love the smell of cow shit." *That's my gal.*

"Here's what you do," he said, trying to hide his disbelief. "Make a list. Put your reasons to marry on one side and your reasons not to marry on the other. Evaluate."

My dad is a scientist; I'm more . . . chaotic. But I did just that on a plane ride. I listed the negatives on one side: religious differences, family pressures, and social and travel differences. On the positive side were: sex, sex (again), fun, sense of style, beautiful, great smile, great laugh, creative, cool career, nurturing, unpretentious, insightful, unusual, understands what's important in life, keeps me from getting too serious, wants the right things out of life, surrounds herself with a varied group of people, isn't intimidated by authority, brings out the best in me, same taste and goals.

So my dad was right. The list was a good idea (the Positives clobbered the Negatives, 20 to 4). Your list will be entirely different from mine, but you may see that the scales are tipped in her favor.

YOUR GIRLFRIEND MAY JUMP THE GUN AND PROPOSE TO YOU. *You don't want to break her heart or disgrace her, but in your heart,* you know you ought to be the one proposing. *(It's that ol' pursuer thing again.)*

If it doesn't matter to you (as it didn't to one buddy of mine), go ahead and say, Yes! If it does, try not to muddle through your reply; it will only humiliate her more. "We were on the banks of the Danube," my friend Louanne said, "and I waited for a really romantic moment, brought out a plastic ring, got down on one knee, and asked him to marry me. He said, 'Aw, come on.' Our plane ride back wasn't so pleasant."

But another friend dumped an indecisive boyfriend (who had wobbled for six years), proposed after only two months to her new boyfriend, and he said, "Yeah! That's great!"

---

91. Listen for "the click."

When I felt my "click," it was as if my cells had rearranged themselves. I suddenly knew this was the woman I must marry, that she'd be just crazy enough to share my absurd trajectory through the universe. I felt flooded with memories—*our* memories. If I didn't marry her, they'd be gone. I nearly proposed that instant, but lying in our mud baths, I said instead, "What's in this mud?!"

"Mud's in the mud," she said.

"I just had a weird thought," I said.

"You always have weird thoughts," she replied.

"No. This one was big weird."

"I'm used to big weird. Tell me!"

But I wasn't ready. I waited another five weeks. "The click" stayed with me. Weird, truly weird. Like a religious conversion.

Like a Red Sox fan saying, "You know, I love the Mets. They're a nice team. I forgive them for Mookie's grounder."

But soon what seemed irrational—marriage—seemed totally rational. I couldn't just skip back to my former thoughts. One instant, it makes no sense. The next, it makes complete sense.

What happened? You've done all your thinking. You can't think about it any more. You're tired of searching for The Perfect Woman. You want to be free. And, against all odds, freedom is . . . with her.

That's one hell of a click.

92. *Even if you're wiped out, make it romantic.*

You've discussed marriage twenty-five billion times. You're living in a ceasefire zone. You're out of ammo. So is she. Then, like a country hoping for permanent peace, you consider the "married" state.

My friend, Frank, was so depleted from the commitment battles that, while reading the morning paper and sipping his coffee, he said, "So . . . are we going?" "Where?" Janice asked between mouthfuls of oatmeal. "Well, you know." "No," she said, not looking up. "Are we, uhm, going to . . . well, you know, get m-m-married? I guess that's what I'm trying to say."

She set down her spoon. "Well, you could be a bit more romantic about it!!" He shrugged and smiled. "Then . . . yes!!" she yelped. "Let's get married!"

Remember that if you propose at Blockbuster Video, her first thought is not going to be, *Oh, I'm going to get married!* Instead, it'll be, "Now for the rest of my life I've got to tell people that I got engaged at Blockbuster Video while deciding between *Serial Mom* and *Basic Instinct.* "

93. *There's no way to make your proposal too romantic.*

You can go completely overboard—and she won't roll her eyes and accuse you of being too sappy.

My friend Woody brought his girlfriend to an abandoned sugar mill at a vacation spot. "It was this wonderful, mossy, overgrown ruin," Erica said wistfully. "He took me to a staircase that he had lined with fresh-cut Bougainvillea. Walking up, I came to a platform where he had made a huge circle of pink, orange, and white flowers. He got on one knee and proposed to me, telling me how I'm beautiful and wonderful and how fun I was and how I'd be a great wife and mother. My heart was pounding. I was in shock. When he took out the ring, it was just so wonderful that I started crying."

Aside from setting some sort of benchmark for romance, Woody was clever to slow down the actual proposal. Give her a chance to realize what's happening.

94. *Don't script your proposal.*

No practicing before the video camera, friends, or a mirror. Shoot straight from the heart and don't worry if you lose your breath or bungle a line or a few words; it will only render your proposal more heartfelt.

I know a guy who wrote eight drafts of an elaborate proposal, left it in his car, forget every word, and went with the minimal, "Will you marry me?"

95. *Consider asking her parents first.*

Most guys don't like asking parents for permission—especially when it's her parents and it's her hand. But if her family is traditional, you'd better play by their rules. Forget your pride; it's for her.

Try not to procrastinate. One friend took his future father-in-law out for eighteen holes of golf for four consecutive days but couldn't find his nerve. His girlfriend said, "Please! No more golf!" But after the proposal, when she discovered his intent, she said to him, "Dad would have held it against you if you hadn't asked him first."

Or, after you propose to her, she may ask you to get her parents' blessing. My wife did (it's what they do in the South). I stared at the phone for minutes and then hung up several times. Finally, I got on the phone and said we were getting married and were out of our minds with happiness and asked would they give us their support.

96. If you're on vacation together, better know in advance if she's going to accept your proposal.

One friend planned an elaborate long weekend away on an island so he could propose. He asked his girlfriend's sister to pack her bag (including passport) and asked his girlfriend to accompany him to the airport to pick up a friend. He surprised her and they boarded a plane. There was only one problem: She'd told him before she wasn't sure yet.

On the plane, she presumed he would propose—and she went to the bathroom and burst into tears. The instant they got to the hotel, he ushered her to their room, poured champagne, took out a ring, fell to his knee, and proposed. Her reply was not a big hit: "Not now. Maybe later?" For the next four days and nights (it was a prepaid vacation; no air changes) they didn't speak to one another. Now they're a great couple, hoping to start a family.

97. Don't worry if your proposal doesn't go exactly as planned.

In this day of been-there, done-that, people want to be different. You hear of proposals while parachuting eight thousand feet. Or guys who propose on televised Lotto broadcasts or while scuba diving, and a shark swims by with a ring taped to its dorsal fin, or by placing an engagement ring in a fortune cookie that's glued back together by Chinese craftsmen.

My friend Paul brought his fiancée-to-be to a romantic dock at sunset. He had loosened the cork on a bottle of wine, scribbled his proposal on a note, wrapped it in plastic, and tied it to the cork. "Have some wine," he said, and tried to hand her the bottle so she'd pull the cork. "No thanks," she said. "Why don't you have some wine?" he said more urgently. "I'm fine," she said. "But why?" he insisted. "I had enough wine with dinner!" she said. By then, the full moon was obscured by a cloud, and he was wondering how he could get her to pull the cork and she was wondering why the hell he wouldn't just propose!

Finally, he said, *"Will you please have some wine!!"* At this point, she needed a drink, so she pulled the cork, spotted the note, and unfolded it. But without the moon, she couldn't read it—so he brought her to a nearby trail light buzzing with bugs, and holding the note close to it, she struggled to read: "You're the most important person in the world to me. Will you marry me?"

It was not quite how he'd pictured it would go, and not quite how she'd pictured it, either. But now it's "perfect."

• • •

98. *Take the plunge.*

I was 100 percent, beyond a doubt, absolutely, resolutely sure that I would propose. Still, I stalled. I felt like a field goal kicker who was watching the goal posts mysteriously move farther away.

Finally, one spring day in the country, the air was perfect and the sky was perfect and she was perfect and everything we did was perfect and I kept telling myself, *OK, dummy, do it! Say the words! Say them!!* I looked into her eyes, began moving my mouth, and said, "You think the Cubs have a chance this year?" My heart was pounding out of my chest. "The Cubs?" she said. "They usually start out strong and get your hopes up and then fall apart, right?"

I thought, *The gods are laughing at me. I have to take the plunge.* A breeze kicked through her hair. So many times, she'd guessed that I was going to propose—and had been wrong. But not this time; she had no idea. I was grilling dinner under a chestnut tree. I stirred the coals, and my hand was shaking. Then, like an idiot, I said, "Back in a flash." I went inside and called my best friend. "I cannot believe what I'm about to do. I'm going to do it. I am. I'm going to ask her." He said, "You're caught in a moment! There will be others! Don't be rash!"

Rash?! Come on! Mount Rushmore was sculpted faster! The Egyptians built pyramids faster! A president had started and finished his term! "Uh-huh . . . right . . . gotcha," I said, setting the phone down.

I dashed outside. And then it happened in a blur. She stared at me in that amazing light. I slipped my hand behind her neck and kissed her. I could feel my heart thumping through my shirt.

I took a breath and said, "You're the most perfect woman ever created, and I'm going to love you forever. Let's be together always—not just this year, not just next. Forever. So, I'd like to know, Will you marry me?"

She pulled back. Her eyes welled with tears and her lower lip was trembling. "You're kidding?"

I shook my head and kissed her again. "Well?"

"Yes . . ." she said. And then we went totally wild, rolling around, hugging, kissing.

And with an unforgettable smile, she tried out her married name.

I liked that. In fact, I loved it.

What had I been afraid of?

Ring Time

99. *Enjoy the twenty-megaton-yoke-being-lifted-off-your-shoulders feeling.*

You now realize that to Propose or Not to Propose had zapped 70 percent of your attention, 90 percent of your energy, and all your sanity for the months and/or years of what could be called the Great Preoccupation. You've unlocked huge portions of your brain that had been otherwise occupied. Now you can think. Now you can relax.

So get used to another sensation: being engaged. Engagement is also a new way of relating to the rest of the world. Your parents. Your job. Your friends. For a while, anyway, you and your fiancée may feel as if you're floating slightly above the rest of the world in a Teflon-coated bubble, where all worldly problems slide right off like the fried egg from a well-oiled frying pan.

OK, it's not all stupendous. You may feel a twinge of remorse, as in missing your former self (read: total control). You may feel a mite jealous of men who are still in the hunt, while you've moth-balled your safari jacket and binoculars. "I felt remorse for the forty-year-old bachelor I'd never be," one buddy said. "It was a sense of foreclosure. I'd never be the established older guy with the young plaything in the short skirt ogling me over my achievements and my ability to tell a waiter how to pour wine or shave truffles."

Some guys *really* feel the relief of having decided. "It was like my brain had been mush for three years," my friend Brian said. Another buddy said, "My life was sane again. I had time. I was glad to push the past away. I even had a dream in which a dark, gangly figure was walking away. The figure was the former me, Mr. Indecisive. Finally gone!"

100. For some of us, we were married the instant we proposed (and she accepted).

If that's the case with you, Congratulations. The ceremony and all the rest are just frosting on the cake.

There's a certain resolve, a calm, that you see in guys who are married before the wedding. It's not that they're in the eye of the storm; for them, there is no storm.

101. The wedding plans may bring out the best—or the worst—in your mother-in-law-to-be.

"We had absolutely zero stress about the wedding because Vicki's mother was so amazing," my friend Howard said. "She handled every detail. Vicki and I did essentially nothing—and the wedding was the greatest day of my life, the best party I've ever been to, a blast. And the most amazing part is, she did all this while going through cancer treatments. It's almost impossible for me to talk about it without getting weepy. I had the most amazing mother-in-law you could imagine."

On the other hand, the wedding plans may send your mother-in-law-to-be into hyperdrive. "Her mother was totally insane," one friend said. "She created a hellish atmosphere." Her mother may pester your fiancée about her weight or offer the services of her plastic surgeon for a little nip-and-tuck. (It can get extreme.)

All this is a preview of how the two of you will work out problems—together. If you take the "It's your mother and your problem" approach, she may wonder who she's marrying.

102. Call your parents and bury the hatchet.
Not everybody is at odds with his or her parents. However, many of us are (including nearly everyone I know). If you spent all of your adolescence and half your adult years gnashing your teeth over your parents, engagement is the time for reconciliation.

Your parents may feel as if they've been hit by a stungun: Their child is no longer their baby. You belong to someone else. From their perspective, it's been a long and rocky road. From one to three, you adored them; from three to thirteen, you put up with them; from thirteen to seventeen, you hated them; from seventeen to when you got engaged, you tried to figure them out. They, too, feel it's probably time to forgive.

I wrote a letter to my parents, saying that a whole lot of water had passed under our bridge and let's let it all flow. I felt liberated from my parents, better able to give myself over to my wife and prepare myself for our future. We all understood that I had a new relationship with my parents. My wife came first.

103. *Stand by the woman you love.*

My friend Paul's parents *really* didn't approve of Joan, his bride-to-be. "I knew they didn't like her, so I was shaking when I called to say I was getting married. My mother screamed and then dropped the phone. I could hear her sobbing and hollering and tossing dishes. My dad was speechless. When my mom got back on the phone, she said she'd never attend our wedding. Later, after she changed her mind and decided to come, she sent a bill, in advance, for her hotel and airfare. That was the last straw. I said, 'Don't bother to come.'"

"That's when Paul became a man," said Joan. "I knew we'd make it as a married couple—and I wasn't quite sure until then. I hated his mother's petty outburst at the time, but it forced us finally to stand up to her."

Two days before the wedding, his parents made peace, flew (at their expense) to a family dinner (the night before the prenuptial dinner), and pretended nothing had happened. The dust settled. All smiles. The mini-soap opera played its final prewedding reel.

How do you stand your ground? During your engagement, there will be many, many times when you will feel placed in the middle—between your mother and your wife. It's this simple: Choose your wife. My friend Hal said his wife had planned a picnic with his parents and had even asked for everyone's favorite foods. At the last moment, his mother called to say she had gotten a reservation at a tough-to-crack, hot-spot restaurant. Hal's wife went berserk—and he had to call his mother and say, "Mom, we'll go there another time. I'll call up and make a reservation for another night—even if it's one month from now." His wife said, "That's when we became a couple. I can't tell you how much it meant to me. I'd always been worried he was a momma's boy. He'd busted out."

104. ***Don't freak if your fiancée reminds you of a great quarterback down by six with 1:42 left on the clock, running a two-minute offense.***

Is there anything finer than watching a great quarterback lead his team eighty-seven yards for the score, eight plays in a minute thirty-one, to take the lead by one with only seven seconds left until time expires? Well, after you've stalled and stalled (and stalled), your fiancée may want to get you into the end zone (the wedding)—spike, slam, bam, boom!—before you change your mind. She's now in a No-Huddle Offense.

I know my fiancée was. Days after we broke the news, she asked me what date I had in mind for the wedding. I scratched my head (somehow, I'd forgotten that I had to do something else besides get engaged). Before I could reply, she said, "June. I've always wanted a June wedding." I said, "June starts in twenty-nine days. Figure three weeks to make the invitations. Three days for postal delivery. That leaves four days for our guests to book airfare and . . ." "OK," she interjected. "July. But not August. That's too close to fall, and I'd never get married in winter." I said July could be hot, and she said, "Not *this* July. *This* July will be cool."

Cut to July 29. 7:00 P.M. The air was so drenched, so steamy, you could pressure-cook an egg *in the air*. At our rehearsal dinner, I sweated through not only my shirt but my sports jacket and even my tie. "Wow, you really know how to sweat, don't you?" one of her relatives said. "Can I get you a towel?" one of the waitresses asked. My hair was wringing wet. *No, I'll just shake off like a dog getting out of a pond. That'll further freak out the relatives on her side.*

OK, so a quick engagement didn't bother me—and it may not bother you. (My feeling was, "Let her have her way. I'm married already.")

But what if you feel it's all going too fast? (It's easy for a com-mitmentphobic man to go into a panic.) Say, "What's the hurry? It's not that I don't want to get married. I'm not having second thoughts. But I'd like to enjoy our engagement."

105. In setting a date, don't take every last family member into account.

Before setting a date, you will be besieged by everyone asking, "Have you set a date?" (Oddly, everyone asks the question in exactly the same tone.)

So, you soon discover that coordinating everyone's agendas is like figuring out the alignments of the earth, sun, and moon for a solar eclipse: very, very complex. Conflicts sabotage the calendar: other people's vacations, sabbaticals, weddings, bar mitzvahs, confirmations, conventions, babies' due dates, golf tournaments, family reunions, weekends to Vegas, World Series games, resodding the lawn (uh-huh: we heard it!). You thought everyone understood that Asking the Question required the collaboration of every cell in your body. You think they'd give you a break, drop everything, and come running. They won't.

Eventually, you stab your finger at a date on the calendar and hope the key players can be there. Present them with the fact and let them adapt.

106. Now that the triumph of nabbing you has worn off, does she seem letdown?

She may suddenly feel exhausted or depressed from having hauled you in like you were a trophy marlin (you may not look half as big and shiny now as you did in the turquoise waters of her mind). You're certainly the same (or better because you're no longer beleaguered by indecision), but she begins to notice some annoying habits. She buys you a new pair of jeans, thinking you'll wear them with loafers to cocktail parties held in celebration of You-the-Couple; instead, you pull them on to clean the gutters and change the wheels on your lawnmower, each time wiping your gunky hands on the front pockets. Or, you're handed a hot, moist napkin at a Japanese restaurant and you wipe not only your hands, but your face, neck, forearms—everywhere but under your armpits. She wants to hide under the table. *Who is this man?! And why did I never notice this stuff before?!*

I'll never forget the look of horror on my fiancée's face when, after a meal of stringy flank steak, I started to floss my teeth with the bottom hem of my T-shirt. Clearly, this is not the sort of thing you dare do during courtship because you're trying to catch her. She thinks, *Do I have to watch this sort of behavior the rest of my life?!*

And she's also sick of everybody telling her, "You must be so happy!" or "You look won-der-ful!" She may not feel she looks so wonderful. She may say, "Am I putting on a few pounds? Be honest. I can handle it. You've got to tell me." Your reply should not be, "Come on, let's rattle off some sit-ups" or "Why don't you buy more flattering pants?" She wants your ear. She's venting her feelings. She's vulnerable, so don't judge, don't pontificate, don't solve, don't call her irrational.

What's going on here? STRESS. What's the solution? Set aside time to get it out in the open. When things go underground during an engagement, they will eventually explode. And then we're talking about Your Anger verses Her Anger. During your engagement, you've got to learn to unplug the phone, turn off the TV, and vent. Take turns. Let each other finish the thought. Once you've let the steam out, you may find yourself laughing at yourself—and then laughing together. That's the twist you're looking for in your engagement.

107. Don't second-guess your early courtship.

Did you sleep together on the first date—not realizing you'd one day marry each other? How about if you did everything in the "wrong" order: you lived together, bought a house, got pregnant, then proposed? Or, you were friends for years, got sloshed, fell into the sack, then realized you were lovers.

I know plenty of couples who did everything in the reverse order—and they're still happily married. "It was ridiculous the way we went about it," one friend said. "We almost got married in Madrid and then didn't. We set up a private wedding on an island and then got lazy. We bought land, built a cabin together, moved in, and a week later, got engaged, called everyone, planned the wedding, discovered she was pregnant (and would be *really* pregnant at the wedding). We started to second-guess ourselves—then we stopped. Big deal! In the end, the service centered on the baby my wife was carrying. The promise felt even more real."

108. Don't look at her bridal magazines.

She's suddenly picking up copies of magazines that could scare you ringless. (*And what's she doing? Filling out a subscription form?*) Worst of all, she's reading these magazines in *bed*—precisely where you don't need to see them. She lobs the magazine to you, and you flip to articles with *dos, don'ts, must-haves, tips, can't-overlooks, don't-forgets, makeovers, perfect-this-and-thats, dream-come-trues.* And it's just chock full of cheesy photos of android wedding couples who seem bloodless, spineless, fightless and—most important—sexless.

Don't worry. Your real-life, out-of-control, dueling-families wedding won't be a bit like those not-a-petal-out-of-place, no-fun fantasy weddings.

109. It's not too early to talk about what you want in day-to-day married life.

Maybe one of you fears shouting and fights and the other fears tedium in the form of washing dishes and clothes. My friend Felicia said, "I want us to be nicer to each other than we are to

friends." Her husband-to-be Patrick said, "I don't want the fighting I saw in my parents." Those two sentiments became the cor-
nerstones for their marriage. "I feared being like my father,"
another friend said. "Nothing I could do was good enough. And
he did nothing but criticize my mother. I didn't want to become
him in my own marriage. I was terrified of becoming a discipli-
narian. And I didn't want to ignore issues until they were unman-
ageable."

What scares you about your day-to-day married life? Chaos?
Too much order? Too much emotion? Lack of emotion? Saving
for the future? Blowing your money now? These are the issues
you must identify for your fiancée so you can begin to handle
them. And then it may be a bit like sketching: You'll add, erase,
highlight, blot. But you never want to lose sight of your original
aims—yours and hers.

110. If she's with you when you're buying her engagement ring and wedding bands, be extra romantic.

Maybe you bought all the rings on your own. Lots of guys have
the fortitude to do it on their own—and to them, I say, Bravo!

But if you're like me—and you want to be sure she likes the
rings she'll be wearing every day for the rest of her life—do it with
flair because she'll remember this moment forever. Don't rush it.
Scope out a few stores, find a salesperson you trust (ha!), set aside
a ring that you think may be right. Then make a date with your
fiancée to see it.

For any man, buying a ring is a surreal moment. My fiancée
and I were about to enter a fancy Manhattan jewelry store, when

I staggered slightly at the prospect. "Don't worry," my bride-to-be said, sensing my trepidation and gently guiding me through the door.

Inside, it was all genteel civility. In the hushed quiet, we selected two reddish gold rings from Birmingham, England, circa 1870. They were thin and elegant and had a deep luster; my fiancée's slipped nicely on her finger. I raised my hand, feeling some trepidation. The first ring didn't fit over my knuckle (I'd broken every one of my fingers playing sports); neither did the second or third. "Let's do this thing right," the salesman said, getting a ring sizer from a drawer. We slipped on one mock ring, then another, until we arrived at the proper size. "This looks like it should go in a bull's nose," I muttered. The salesman assured me that my newly sized ring would be perfect. "Let's inscribe them," my fiancée said. "Forever," I whispered. *Precisely the concept that had held me back for four years.*

Outside, we walked excitedly to another store for the engagement ring. My fiancée held my elbow and snuggled close; clearly, this was a peak moment for her—and, I had to admit, for me, too.

A saleswoman greeted us and brought out the ring I'd selected. "Oh!" my fiancée sighed. "It's beautiful." And it was already hers in her mind. If it fit—and it did. "Don't you want to see others?" I asked. "No," she said. "There's another ring over there . . ." "Nope. This is it. It's mine. It's perfect."

As always, I envied her decisiveness. The day before, when I had selected the ring, the saleswoman had asked me, "How much do you hope to spend?" At that time, "hope" and "spend" seemed like polar opposites, but here, today, with my fiancée's eyes glimmering, I understood the concept. (I'm not saying you ought to break the bank, but get a ring that will make her happy.)

Light a candle that night, make love with your fiancée. Make love with your rings on — just once. That ought to send you both to high heaven.

DON'T GO RING CRAZY. *Suddenly, you hear a lot about cut, clarity, color, and carat weight. But your head is already spinning with diamond shapes: radiant, princess, heart, pear, marquise, brilliant, emerald, oval, trillion, quadrillion. And diamond colors. And terms like the table, girdle, pavilion, and culette. And rules like spending two months' salary on the ring. Aghhh!!! You're thinking:* Please God, just don't let it be a fake!

The key is to buy with your heart. It should feel almost like fate when you find the right ring.

---

111. No, the wedding is not for you.
It's for the parents and in-laws. Oh, hell, it's for her mother and yours — in that order.

My wife's mother invited us for tea so we could give our input on the wedding. This seemed to me an exceptionally open gesture. "So," she said in her deep southern drawl, "tell me what kind of weddin' you have in mind?"

"Casual," I said.

"Casual," she repeated as if she had never heard the word.

"Yeah. How about a country band and barbecue? Grilled chicken, corn, tomatoes, watermelon, coleslaw, beer, and wine. Nothing fancy. And instead of everyone standing around and just talking during the day, how about we organize sailboats and three-legged races. You know: fun."

She stared ahead coldly and patted down her hair.

I shifted gears. "OK. How about a Tuscan-style wedding? An Italian peasant band parades around, and we have long tables with billowing white table clothes and carafes of wine and square pizzas and olives and pasta and a meat dish. Like something out of a Fellini movie."

My fiancée piped in, "I like the Tuscan idea more."

My mother-in-law-to-be didn't say a word. Then: "I see poached salmon. Dill sauce. Champagne. Elegant. Restrained but elegant. You'll wear a blue blazer and white pants. She'll wear my wedding dress."

White pants? I saw grass stains, red wine stains, and dog-slobber stains. OK, I would surrender my Wedding-as-Square-Dance for the salmon, but champagne? Couldn't I bargain for Rolling Rock in lock-neck bottles? "Isn't champagne awfully extravagant?" I offered.

"Champagne gives me a headache, Mama," my fiancée said.

My soon-to-be mother-in-law delivered a look that said, *There'll be champagne, or there won't be a weddin'*. And then I realized: It wasn't *our* wedding; it was *her* daughter's wedding. I knew I'd better just go with the flow.

If you want it to be yours and your fiancée's, plan it and pay for it yourselves. Then invite all the family with the explicit understanding: Bring us your dancing shoes, but not your ideas.

Otherwise, let them have their day.

112. *You will want to consider eloping.*

When everyone is driving you and your bride-to-be batty, one of you is bound to blurt, "Let's just run down to city hall." You both know it's the rational thing to do. By pocketing the wedding funds, you could make a down payment on a home with a yard and a dog with a bone. But something drives you forward. You're going to be Indiana Jones reaching for the golden chalice, knowing full well that an enormous boulder will come rolling your way and you'll have to jump into a snake pit of writhing cobras.

Why do you continue?

Because somewhere in your collective unconscious, you know *all this* is forging a stronger relationship between you and your bride. You're learning to handle family. You're learning to negotiate. You're getting a sneak preview of the ups and downs of marriage's roller-coaster ride. Somehow, you know all these skills will come in handy.

113. *Stay out of the War Room as much as possible.*

A room in your mother-in-law's home will be given over to the hyperplanning of the wedding. Women will comprehend this revered space, but to you, it will appear as absurd as the War Room in *Dr. Strangelove.* What will you find there? Lists of guests in three categories: accepted, declined, and too damned lazy to return the reply card in the self addressed stamped envelope.

There will be pages of circles and rectangles (representing tables) and mock-ups of seating plans. There will be lists of effusive, seemingly inedible food combinations, such as morsels of Egyptian figs with blood orange essence floating over a pool of pomegranate reduction.

In the War Room, people will argue strategy. "I never should have invited your aunt and uncle from Cleveland," your future mother-in-law says. Your fiancée counters, "But you have to. He's your brother." "Well, he's an alcoholic and womanizer who wrapped his Lexus around a locust tree, and she's a lazy, gin-guzzling bridge player with viper friends and foul manners." But after a robin's egg blue box arrives in the mail from the aforementioned relatives, the previous allegations will be dropped.

This room may start out sedate, but by Week Eleven, it's a place of screaming, hawking, vulturous cries. It's not for you.

114. Know your wedding responsibilities.

So what do you have to do? A few months before, you've got to buy your attire (or make plans to rent it), plan your honeymoon, help with invitations, help plan the rehearsal dinner, hem and haw over the guest list, hire the officiant, hire music or entertainment, help your bride-to-be with thank-you notes (the gifts are already to the ceiling) and nibble the endless catered samples. A few weeks before, get your marriage license, be sure your rings are back from the jeweler (forever is one word), and finalize the honeymoon plans. The week before, be sure your nails, teeth, and hair look ... human, your honeymoon bags are packed, and tips are ready. The day of the wedding, shave without nicking your chin, dress without perspiring, and get to the ceremony an hour in advance.

So all this doesn't get too mundane, do something silly like say "I love you" to your fiancée in a exotic languages. (Zulu, *Ngiyakuthanda*; Tahitian, *Ua Hre Vau la oe*; Eskimo, *Nagligivaget*; Polish, *Kocham Cie*; Klingon, *Qabang*.)

Meanwhile, just pray you don't get a pimple on the tip of your nose on your wedding day.

115. Buy a bridal gift.

It's an old tradition—and if you have a traditional gal, she's expecting one. What is a bridal gift? It's a gift you're giving her to show her yet again that She's The One. (My friend Howard said, "I thought I was the gift. But I got one anyway.")

My gift for my fiancée was a big hit: I bought her a case of wine that wouldn't be ready to drink for years. (The message of the gift was, *We'll be together forever*.) Every time we opened a bottle, we thought back to way back when, before we were married. Romantic stuff.

116. Make your mark.

My fiancée's mother said it was a southern tradition that the groom pick up the tab for music at the wedding. (Highly debatable, but I didn't call all my southern sources to verify.) I took it as an opportunity to indicate *my* personality.

I telephoned my downstairs' neighbor from my bachelor apartment, the lead tenor from *Phantom of the Opera*, a man whose operatic voice lessons had lifted through my floorboards for years. ("Not: 'La.' More: 'Laaaaa!'") He looked like Pavoratti. And when he sang Puccini as my bride walked down the aisle, I thought everyone would topple over from crying so hard.

Use your imagination.

117. Make your voice heard when selecting invitations.

For some reason, selecting the wedding invitations really flips guys out. The choices are endless. You have engraving, embossing, thermography, offset printing, and calligraphy; corrugated, mylar, moiré, linen, laid, vellum, cotton, jacquard, and parchment; and then twelve trillion typefaces, each of which has a precise meaning to the control freaks at Wedding Central.

And then there's the totally bizarre rule: No everyday numbers (as in 1, 2, 3, 4). Instead, it's "Fourteen Ninety-two and a Half Sunrise Circle East (at Route One Thirty-Three)" and "Half past seven o'clock" on "March, the twenty-ninth, two thousand and . . ." And what do we make of those weird brethren, "Request the pleasure of your company" and "request the honor of your presence?" And what's with these itty-bitty response cards and envelopes, inner and outer envelopes, and the minimalist blank cards? By the time you're done with maps and hotel information cards and rain-instruction cards and ceremony programs, you'd think the entire enterprise is intended to strike terror in a man's heart.

And then I got it: The invitation is an emblem of You-the-Couple, the first indication of Who You Will Become. Granted, those no-numbered invitations don't bother most people. But to me they felt as overdone as Michael Jackson's face, and I suggested that we hand-write the invitations ourselves.

It felt real and homespun, and everyone commented on "how different" we were as a couple. (We felt like mavericks.) But writing out your own invitations is good only for small weddings—or you'll be icing your arm like Pedro Martinez after he whiffed sixteen batters.

118. Invite all your parents' current spouses.

One parent may lobby for an exclusion of an ex's spouse. This is clear-cut retribution (the parent is saying, "We'll play out our *war* over *your* wedding").

But I know weddings where *all* the ex-spouses attended—with their kids, from marriages one through four (where's the Astrodome when you need it?). There was bad behavior preceding the wedding weekend (bitching, back stabbing). sBut the actual weekend went off without a hitch. Howareya's and   nicetoseeya's. And then, amazingly: temporary reconciliation. Why? Because the love between you and your bride intoxicates those around you.

The open-arms policy is best.

119. Don't freak out over the stratospheric cost of her wedding dress.

You will hear amazing justifications for the wild expenditure. My fiancée claimed, "I'll dye it black after the wedding so I can wear it *all the time*." Another buddy heard, "I'll hem it to midthigh, and it'll be perfect for parties."

Just say, "Uh-huh. Sure."

120. Register for wedding gifts.

My fiancée dragged me to a huge department store so we could register, but I froze in front of the antique fish knifes. "Can I talk with you a moment?" I said, pulling my fiancée away from the stare of the saleswoman. "I hate these things. They look like something married people would get." I then realized I wanted to *be* married without *looking* married. "What would you rather have?" my bride-to-be whispered. "A kayak," I said. She just stared. "His and hers parabolic skis—as curvy as you," I said. No response. "How 'bout Fiesta Ware?" Perfect.

For a while, we used the plates only on special occasions; now, we use them every day.

P.S. Even if you do register, you'll still get the occasional hand-me-down gift, like the barf-colored ceramic heart with tiny flowers pasted to it, stuffed into a shoe box, packed with old newspaper. You'll know this was from a couple who didn't register and wanted to pawn the mistake they got off on you.

121. No excuses. Go on a honeymoon.

A friend of mine said to his fiancée, "I'm on a roll at work, and we can *always* go on a honeymoon." She was too stunned to speak. He continued: "The timing is really bad. I'm in the middle of a deal. It's important. You understand, don't you?"

No. She didn't. (She wanted to gouge his eyes out.) And here's why: You can't really go on a honeymoon later because you'll never really be newlyweds again. A honeymoon is not just another vacation! This is about setting priorities. It's about romance. (Something our world could use a bit more of.)

Eventually, my friend took his bride to France—but it wasn't the same (a fact she still reminds him of).

122. *Talk about honeymoon expectations—beforehand.*
Now is not the time for top-secret plans. Go over every aspect of your itinerary together.

And don't get bamboozled by your travel agent. My travel agent hadn't listened to my request for a lazy vacation in an exotic place with nothing much to do (but be romantic). The itinerary she sent was more hectic than a presidential hopeful doing ten states in nine days. (It featured visiting a dragon, and my fiancée said, "I don't want to see any *dragon* on my honeymoon!") I fired the travel agent and got someone who could listen.

123. *Get in top shape or, for the rest of your life, you'll hear, "Who's that chubby guy with the three chins in your wedding photo?"*
There's arguably no photo that will haunt you like a wedding photo. It will stare out at you from a piano top or fireplace mantle for the rest of your life.

Only weeks before my wedding, I realized it was time to take off some pounds—and I got phobic about the wedding-pictures-to-be. After weeks of oatmeal (no milk, no honey, just cranberry juice), lots of carrots and celery sticks, rice crackers, salads with lemon wedges and tons and tons of grapefruit and tomatoes (the Groom's Diet), I looked like a lean, mean marriage machine.

124. *Don't wait until the last moment to understand the difference between premarital jitters and legitimate fears.*

Rattling through every guy's brain are horror stories of guys who couldn't get the signals straight until the final hour.

I saw the catcher from my weekly softball game, at his own wedding, dressed in his tux, behind the church with his best man, smoking a joint, taking a Valium, and saying, "She's over two hours late. Should I go through with this?" His best man said, "She's getting her dress altered. She got stuck in traffic." "That's not the point," the groom said. "I want out." His best man responded, "You're right. You're too nervous. Let's bolt." My friend said, "I'll give her ten more minutes. If she's not here, I'm gone." She showed up and they got married. (They were divorced three years later.)

Another: My cousin watched in dismay as his childhood buddy broke down sobbing in a back room (with an organ humming and guests whispering about a delay in the wedding). "I can't do it! I can't go through with it!" he wailed. He got up, wiped himself off and walked down the aisle. (He and his wife were divorced six years later.)

But the story that really got me panicked was my friend Ricky's. Ricky had a horrendous wedding weekend of bad vibes and a clearer picture that the future wouldn't work. Then, after intense discussions that involved his fiancée, her family, and the priest, he called off his wedding at 5:00 A.M. on the morning it was to take place. (He later married the right woman, and they have a great life together.)

Another guy who called off his wedding at the eleventh hour

told me, "I couldn't sleep. I was going through with it because I thought I had to. I knew it would be a disaster later down the road for both her and me. I did what I had to do: called it off. Then years later, without trepidation, I got married. Now, I've got a wife and two kids and I'm totally content."

Think long and hard, but don't wait 'til the eleventh hour.

125. Be prepared for one terrifying, wide-awake night.
Don't say or do anything rash. Don't jostle her awake and send lethal tremors through your engagement. Wait until morning. It's a cliché (but all clichés have some truth to them): Things will seem less dramatic in the light of day.

You slowly learn that you can't blurt out everything you think without damaging the woman you love (and ultimately your relationship).

DON'T FLIP OUT WHEN A MARRIED BUDDY SAYS, "IN MARRIAGE, YOU LEARN THAT SEX ISN'T EVERYTHING." Most of the time, you hear from single guys that they have sex four times a week. (Bad enough: you feel like an underperformer.)

But what really freaks you out is the opposite. You're having a beer with a guy who's been married a decade, when he says in a low voice, "My wife and I rarely have sex. I know this is hard to explain, but I don't miss it. First, the adventure went. Then, it became routine. Finally, it just petered out. I can't be bothered. At best, we have sex two times in one week and then not at all for three or four months." You nod and smile—but inside, you're freaking out. You realize that nobody but a fool gets married for sex. But while you've ruled out sex with other women, you've also been assuring yourself that you'll have tons of sex with your future wife.

Tell her that sex is the barometer. While you may not have needed to discuss sex during your early courtship, you may have to from now on. How do you talk about sex? Just say it. Don't be vague. Don't use codewords. Don't wrap your thought in a bunch of gobbledygook. Be sure she understands your wants and needs, and vice versa. Teach her what you like (in plain English), and you're more likely to get it. (And vice versa.). And always be complimentary. Say, "I adore it when you do ____ to me. You're so good at that." It shouldn't be any more embarrassing than saying, "I'd like more hot sauce on my taco."

All this goes a long way toward ensuring that sex doesn't slip out of your marriage.

126. God has a very strange sense of humor.

An engaged buddy was on a trans-Atlantic business trip, minding his own business, sitting in his seat on the runway when an Amazing Creature charged down the aisle for her seat. "You could feel every single man on the plane praying that she'd have the seat beside him. And, as it turned out, she squiggled in beside me.

"My first reaction was, *Why did this never happen when I was single—when I was desperate to meet a woman? Huh? God, are you listening?*

"She fell asleep with her head on my shoulder. It was surreal. In the morning, at baggage claim, she said, 'So, you want to share a cab?'

"I said, 'N-n-no, thanks.'"

You may have your own version of this story. Another friend recounted how the wedding photographer's cute assistant slinked into a photo meeting in cut-offs and a tight T-shirt and tilted her head at him as if to say, *Silly! Why are you getting married?*

The answer is: You'll always be tempted: You're a guy!

127. *Beware of the old-fashioned bachelor party.*

Sometime before I was to be married, a buddy called me up to organize my bachelor party. I said I'd rather go to a blues bar or a Yankees game. I'd once been to a friend's bachelor party when his bride-to-be peeked into the room (at just the wrong moment), and shrieked, "It's off! The whole fucking thing is off!" The marriage took place a few wounded days later, but it left an impression on me.

"You've got my word," my friend said. "It will be a harmless night of cards, booze, stogies, and a dirty flick or two. A night to remember."

What struck me about my own bachelor party was precisely its forgetability. There was a vomit-inducing combo of drinking and burping and oily foods and chest pounding and antimarriage jokes. I felt as if I were attending my own funeral, a weird mix of Barnum and Bailey and primal screaming.

But suddenly, there's a choice in bachelor parties. The golf weekend. Skiing bumps. Shooting rapids. Wine tastings. Scotch tastings. Cigar tastings. Even spa night for the boys. The best bachelor party I ever attended was for my cousin in California: boogie boarding, followed by clam bake, followed by a bonfire, songs, and a night swim.

Ask yourself the following questions so you can help your buddies create a bachelor party you'll enjoy—and one that won't haunt you. Do you really want to get stinking drunk? Or do you hope to set a tone among the men who will attend your wedding? Is your fiancée the type who doesn't mind you having a night of debauchery? Or would she totally freak out if you shared the backseat of a limo with a high-priced call girl in nothing but an overcoat? All this will help ensure that you get the bachelor party you want.

128. So you'll be less nervous, make a checklist of what to wear on the big day.

Write down everything, from underwear to handkerchief to socks to shoes—or you'll be standing in a dressing room, staring down at your feet, and wondering if anybody can lend you a pair of shoes.

Try on your clothes (in front of your bride-to-be) a week before the big day. Now walk. Sit. Now, shake, boy. (It's good practice; during you're wedding, you'll feel a bit like a dog doing tricks.)

Think of every detail. Sandpaper the bottoms of your new shoes so you don't slip on marble church steps and feel like a clown. Practice tying your new tie. Snap the cummerbund. Shake hands with your wife to be sure the cummerbund won't pop off (don't laugh: I saw it happen—not on me).

Go ahead. You may now kiss the bride.

129. Pack your honeymoon bag at least three days before your wedding.

Those last frantic days before the wedding, with guests calling from airports needing last-minute lifts, is not the time to pull things together. Make a list of stuff you'll need. Think of everything. If it's sunny, think sun protection. If it's humid, think mosquitoes. If it's mountains, think layers. If it's beach, think books (you'll have time to read, too). Place all of it in a suitcase and close it. Now lift it (if your arm is about to pull out of its socket, simplify). Pack a carry-on bag with essentials, since your bag could easily end up in a neighboring island or distant destination. Your bride will admire your prescience.

If you want to be a real hero, ask your bride-to-be to show you what she's packed. (You'll be carrying her bag, too, but that doesn't mean you have editing power.) "Don't look at that!" she'll say of a lacy thing. "That's a surprise."

She's right; mystery is the name of that game.

130. Don't have sex with your fiancée for two weeks before the wedding.

If you and your fiancée are virgins, I imagine your wedding night will be something you'll remember for a good, long while.

But if you're like most of us, you have a choice: Forget sex on the honeymoon night and invite all your out-of-town relatives up to your room for a night of partying (not my choice, bro!) or make the sex special.

But it's not so easy to do something new after you've gone through a rosy period of having sex many times per week for months on end. My bride-to-be had a plan: She sent me to a road-side motel for the nights preceding our wedding. Her logic was that I'd hunger for her like a panting, sex-crazed virgin. "Brilliant," all her female friends agreed.

I wasn't sure. But it worked.

131. *Don't be mortified by the prospect of a mini-melting-pot wedding weekend.*

I had been. I guessed my wife's family had never spent so much time with liberal, Democratic, midwestern Jews of Russian and Lithuanian descent. And I supposed my family had never spent so much time with southern, conservative, Republican Episcopalians of Welsh and German descent.

In my mind, all my relatives shopped at Loehman's (not true) and hers looked like Ralph Lauren ad models (not true). I considered sending a handbook to my relatives with instructions like (1) Don't finish what's on your plate—especially if it's delicious and you're still hungry. (2) Don't talk about the lightest matzah balls you ever ate. (3) Do talk about renting houses on Nantucket, Martha's Vineyard, and Sea Island. (4) Do ask for a Pimm's Cup and mention the best cricket match you ever saw. (5) Gefilte fish? No. Fly fishing? *Yes!*

But I could relax—as I suggest you do—if you have a mini-melting-pot on your hands because everyone is on your side. They want you to succeed. They want you to walk down the aisle. And when they ask you, "So, do you hunt?" it's best (if you don't hunt) to turn it around and say, "No, my people are fruit and nut gatherers." I liked it when my wife's wild, eighty-seven-year-old great-aunt (who still wore a sexy black slip when she got a physical from her handsome young doctor) said, "I'm so glad you're part of the family. We've got a Turk, a lesbian . . . and now we've got a Jew." She meant it; it was sweet and heartfelt.

If you're a card-carrying, red-blooded commitmentphobe, you're probably panicked that Something May Happen. You envision heated arguments at wedding tables over gun control legislation, birth control, the pope, or the death penalty. None of that will happen. (Anybody who discusses the death penalty at a wedding ought to be taken away by the men in white.) But there's more: Ultimately, you and your bride set the tone. If you project love, the weekend will turn into a veritable love fest.

Even if you're like me, and you adore huge crowds (I once saw the Dalai Lama in Central Park in the morning, a Yankee's game in the afternoon, and a rock concert at night), you may not like having people staring at *you*. The wedding weekend may still be, as it was for me, a nearly hallucinogenic shot of love and encouragement you'll never forget.

PREPARE FOR THE COUNTDOWN. Time will speed up. Your heart will race as you realize: In one hour, I'll be married. In thirty-four minutes, I will be married.

Know it's normal to feel overwhelmed—but you don't want to go into fight-or-flight mode. Try various relaxation techniques. Wiggle your toes in your shoes (that gets you out of your head and into your body). If you're in a seated position, never stand up quickly (or the blood will rush out of your heart, and you'll feel faint). Instead, tuck in your pelvis and count to ten as you stand. Try long exhales. Find your center. Pull in your gut and get in the sports-ready position (knees slightly bent, feet shoulder width, arms bent at a forty-five-degree angle).

---

132. Expect to feel out of body during the vows.

You've seen so many weddings on TV and in the movies that there's a tendency to float out of your shoes and watch your wedding from above. *Who's moving lips are those? Oh, yeah, he's the guy who's marrying me. Who's that guy with the slightly lost, nervous look? Oh, yeah, that's me.*

I once saw a groom go seriously off the deep end. During the vows, he began biting his cheek so he wouldn't burst into giggles. At first, the minister tried to ignore the chuckles. The bride shot him the I'll-kill-you-do-you-hear-me? KILL-YOU! glares. But by the time the minister asked, "Do you take this woman to be your lawfully wedded bride?" the groom was doubled over and the minister had to say, "I take that as 'yes.'"

I can see how it happened to this poor guy. Occupy your mind with something other than what's at hand. The magnitude is too great for some of us—and that's OK.

Even if you've attended tons of weddings, it's different when it's you standing up front in the fancy shoes. When you're asked to put a ring on her finger and receive one on your own, it *might* be a transcendent moment for you, but it's *certainly* going to be one for her. Watch her gleam.

"I've been more riveted by many seesaw, eight-to-seven base-ball games than I was by my own wedding," one buddy said. "But my wife was glowing!"

Of course, you may zoom off into the stratosphere. One friend recounted how he'd never met his wife's father (who had died the previous year)—and didn't, quite frankly, expect much from the ceremony. They were married under a tree her father had planted in their backyard. "Standing there, under that tree, I sensed his presence. It was as if I understood a new part of her."

133. There may be a moment of clarity during the ceremony.
Mine came during the breaking of the glass (a Jewish tradition). The rabbi explained that it symbolized the destruction of the temple—but to me, as my foot came crashing down on the glass (wrapped in a napkin), it was all about shattering my bachelorhood.

I hadn't practiced crushing glasses, and I worried that my foot might not hit the glass head on. What if it squiggled free like a loose pigskin on a failed field goal?

But I laid into this one, and the glass shattered to smithereens. Gone. Kaput.

Amid the cheers, I wanted to raise my arms à la Rocky! I wanted to whoop! Out with the old! In with the new!

134. Don't network at your wedding.
"Our wedding was one big business opportunity for him," my friend Joyce said of her new husband. "Nick was really work-ing the crowd, pushing for favors, closing deals. It was awful. He was slapping palm and schmoozing and cutting points on real

estate closings. I watched in horror and wondered who I married."

Tune in to your new bride. If someone hands you a cellular phone with a business question, tell them you have an emergency: You're getting married (say it in earshot of your bride).

135. *"From this moment forth" starts the instant you leave the wedding.*

Maybe the wedding was more an expression of your mother-in-law's taste than your own. Fine. But when you drive off, it's your gig. Your life. Your style.

My wife and I took off down the bumpy driveway in what was now "our" battered white Bronco. "Well, that was wild," I said. I stopped and kissed her, then we headed toward our immediate future—a ramshackle inn, about a fifteen-minute drive over a ridge. My choice of a wedding-night hotel had *not* been a big hit with my mother-in-law. ("I can't imagine what you're thinking," she said.) But the second we pulled into the big dirt drive, I knew my choice had been right. It was an expression of where I felt my wife and I were going—not somebody else's idea. There was a huge grain silo and an old farmhouse, and the sky was ablaze with lit clouds, and it seemed unpretentious and the opposite of champagne.

We felt free.

HAVE A MIDNIGHT SNACK READY. Maybe you and your bride didn't have a chance to take a bite of food. Now the hotel kitchen is closed. There's not a store for miles. The minibar offers four-

dollar M & Ms, five-dollar pretzels, and six-dollar salted peanuts. She shoots you a "Great provider you are" look.

Come on, now. It's your honeymoon night! Have some aphrodisiac foods on hand. Strawberries. Smoked salmon. Or stimulants like chocolate.

One friend went oyster crazy. "I thought of Casanova, who was known to down fifty oysters while bathing with a beautiful babe. I thought of a Dead Head telling me that zinc increased testosterone and sperm count. And I realized, I want oysters on my wedding night!"

If you're not into oysters, at least get an extraordinary bottle of wine.

---

136. Give her a family heirloom on your honeymoon night.

You may feel tapped out by now, and you might loathe (as I did) the superficiality of most gifts you've already received. But a family heirloom is different. This is the biggest day of her life so far, and you want to connect her with the past, and particularly, your family's past. Ask your mother or grandmother about jewelry, maybe earrings or a necklace. Or an old frame with a photo of you and her. Or a musical instrument. Or some quirky item that meant something to you as a kid—not your baseball cards.

The note you write will be just as important (and I don't care how messy your handwriting, don't do the tacky thing and have a calligrapher do more of that God-awful scribbly script). Tell her she's now part of your family.

Present her with your gift and note soon after you enter your honeymoon room.

GO LIGHT ON THE WEDDING POSTMORTEM. Few can resist dissecting a party or second-guessing it until it reminds you of a frog after a high school anatomy class. Don't go there.

The wedding was what it was. Yeah, it took a ton of planning and it was over in a flash—and if you knew then what you know now. One friend took a serious nosedive after the wedding. "It was all arranged to suit my parents' social obligations! It was all for show! A display of money!" However, his wife said, "He-llo? That's what it was for them! But we had a great time! And we're married!"

Your wedding doesn't have to be the happiest day of your life—or hers.

---

137. Spend time alone with your bride before you dive into bed.

You can't just switch gears from the We're So Happy! moment of the wedding to the Hey, Baby, Wanna Get Down Tonight? moment of your honeymoon night.

But now is not the time to numb yourself. You want to remember every detail. My wife suggested we take a walk down a twisting country road. (My immediate reaction was, *I'd never have thought of that! There's her True North again.*) The hills were covered in mist, so only nearby tree trunks were visible; we held hands and felt incredibly couple-ish. I hadn't anticipated any of this and realized that I'd been so focused on the wedding weekend and the honeymoon, that I hadn't planned on an intermediate, transition period.

I'm not sure how far we walked or when we came back, but when we closed the creaky door to our tiny room, with its faded wallpaper and leaded windows, there was a sense of anticipation. A lamp in the corner cast a yellow glow. The house was hushed. The whole experience was dreamlike in a way the actual wedding hadn't been. (Vivid sex description deleted by author's wife.)

138. Don't flip out if you don't have the big bang.

A buddy of mine admitted, "I was so stressed out about the whole wedding thing, I cried. I wailed, 'I hope our lives will be as good as I'd planned them to be.' So, there we were, in our honeymoon room, and my new wife was consoling me and telling me everything would be all right and that we ought to just go to sleep. She poured me a brandy and I steadied myself, but it's not as though we could have segued from my crying spasms into roaring sex."

A big wedding is not necessarily the perfect preamble to sure-fire sex. Your head may be spinning from details or you may be emotionally spent or your feet may ache so much from tearing up the dance floor that all you want is a good foot massage. "Our wedding lasted until 1 A.M., and Vicki always likes to be the *last* to leave," my friend Howard said. "By the time we got to our hotel, we were totally exhausted. And it was fine."

NEVER RIDICULE YOUR WIFE'S OR YOUR MOTHER-IN-LAW'S ROMANTIC GESTURES. *My mother-in-law took a piece of our wedding cake and placed it in our freezer, explaining we'd eat it on our first anniversary. I wanted to say, "Yeah. It's going to be sufficiently freezer-burned to taste like Styrofoam." (Wisely, I kept my mouth shut.)*

A year later, it was unspeakably inedible—and I waited for my wife to say (as she nearly choked), "Mama, that was so sweet of you."

139. Write thank-you notes to your parents and in-laws.

Get these two notes off on the plane and mail them upon your arrival.

Now is the moment to thank our parents not only for their participation in the wedding but for making you who you are and preparing you for life. (If your letter isn't a tearjerker, you've failed.) Let them know you appreciate their guidance—and you'll do everything to make them proud. (OK, be a little sappy.) Tell them how the first day or days of married life have been (obviously, don't give them the X-rated version).

I don't care how you fall over yourself thanking your in-laws for the wedding, if they don't get a note that is postmarked within a few days of the wedding, they'll start grumbling about Their Ungrateful Louse of a Son-in-law. In this note, you want to reassure your new ma and pa that you'll take care of their baby.

Reminder: a crackly thank-you telephone call with steel drums pounding in the background does not excuse you from a heartfelt note.

140. Take advantage of your newly married status.

Not to be a freeloader, but what the hell is wrong with getting an upgrade from coach to first class or from a standard room with a springy mattress to a penthouse suite with acres of bed?

Here's how it's done. Walk up to the most friendly looking attendant at the front desk. Smile and say hello (reading the attendant's name off the tag). Explain that you and your bride (she smiles and blushes) are on your honeymoon and you'd be forever appreciative if an upgrade were possible. You're dressed nicely. You look tip-worthy. When you get your upgrade, get the name of the hotel manager and write a recommendation letter later. Tip generously.

A bottle of champagne or a basket of fruit may even be delivered to your room in half an hour.

141. But sometimes adversity will throw things into perspective. My bride and I were far, far away in a hut with a thatched roof. I lay awake listening to the breeze and took long walks in the moonlight, down to the sea, where everything felt new and I could hardly believe I'd waited so long to get married.

We rented a moped and explored our little island. We rode through little villages and rice terraces. When we'd stop, kids would gather round, and I'd imagine my new wife as a mother one day.

But a week into our honeymoon, I woke up at 2 A.M. with a fever and a throbbing near my pancreas. Delirious, I was rushed to a remote hospital, where workers were mopping disinfectant on the floors. Tests indicated that I had typhoid. I wondered if I'd die. I told my wife how happy I was that I'd married her, how stupid I'd been with my indecision, and how sorry I was to have put her through it all. I felt a fool. If I'd been *this* sick in a foreign land, with nobody to care for me, I'd have been alone.

For the next week, back at our hut, I lay in a hammock and gazed at clouds and drank milk and took medication. I said to my bride, "I can't believe this is happening! This is our honeymoon! I'm wrecking it for you!" She said, "Shh . . . this is what marriage is all about." And that's when I learned "for better or worse, 'til death do us part" isn't so bad. I stared at her. She was so beautiful. We imagined our future together. We drifted. We listened to birds and waves. In a weird way, it was almost fortunate that I got sick. We'd done many things during our dating years (movies, ballgames, trips)—but never typhoid. We reached somewhere deeper than a cheery honeymoon would have provided. We'd bonded.

When I finally recovered (we extended the honeymoon), I felt transformed—and *really* married.

And totally, unbelievably, in love.

Starting Out—and Staying Committed

142. Don't get freaked out by everyone telling you, "Marriage takes work."

All the longtime married couples tell you about work and marriage, marriage and work. You think, *Long-term commitment sounds like a pretty tough deal. I give up adventure and get work? Something's wrong with this picture.*

Too sober! Here's what you have to keep in your marriage: imagination, romance, passion, sex, surprises, gifts, dirty stories, slipping hands on thighs under dinner tables, and lots of "You're amazing—and I'm so lucky to be going through life with you."

When things get rough (and they will), remember that laughter will get you back on track. The "work" of marriage is creating time to have fun and connect.

143. Ignore everyone who tells you, "Marriage is a 50–50 percent proposition."

Good news: It's bunk.

You'll learn very quickly that marriage is *not* like figure skating: You, the Shiny Couple, dancing along the ice in perfect unison, smiles pasted on your faces, blades cutting into the ice, wife spiraling into the air, husband effortlessly catching her, followed by Big Artificial Smile, deep bow to the judges, and *ta-das* north, south, east, and west!

Ah, no. Even after a few months, you discover that life is almost never easy for two people at once. There may be weeks or months when one of you will hold up the other. Better to think of marriage as alternately 75–25 percent, then 25–75 percent. Later on, if one of you can't get any traction in your work or life, it may even be 95–5 percent for weeks or months. Rarely does it ever balance at the magical 50–50 percent.

Don't ever bother to keep score; it all averages out in the end.

144. Get over the first hurdle.

You hear all the time about the beginning of marriage being hell on earth. (It shouldn't be.) Why is that?

Because you're grafting two lives together. And because you imagined every moment would be magical. She's your dream girl. She's gonna fix everything. All fights shall cease. Peace on earth. Just cows in pastures chewing their cuds and looking up as if to say, "They're in love."

Instead, you feel buried in an avalanche. You've got to add her name to everything, from the bank account to the insurance policy. You've got heaps of gifts you can't stand. You've got piles of thank-you notes waiting to be written. You've got stacks of proof sheets and sampler wedding photos and a pushy photographer nudging you to decide (buy the negatives so you can fulfill the endless—and ever-changing—orders from your families). You've got your wife's wedding dress, which she wants to preserve so her daughter (her *what?!*) can wear it thirty years hence . . . and she's already wondering how to mummify the lacy thing. You've got a meeting with a lawyer to draw up wills, and despite his ungodly rate per hour, you notice a hint of bourbon under his Certs.

Here's what we did to fight this: We celebrated every night. We dashed home from work and put a little extra *umph* into our dinners and danced around our living room and felt . . . lucky. Say to your wife, "Can you believe we've been married two weeks!" Or ". . . two months!"

Keep it romantic.

145. Learn the basics of marital communication.

(1) *When you're criticizing, begin sentences with "I feel," rather than "You are," or "You always do."* There's a huge difference between "You're not paying attention to what I'm saying!" and "I feel as though we're not listening to each other." The first statement is like a jab in the sternum; the second distributes the weight over both your shoulders.

(2) *Don't be vague.* It's easy—but not effective—to circle an issue endlessly like a plane without a runway. It's better to be precise. Say what you mean. "I hate when you do that!" means less than "I feel like you're leaving me hanging when you're late and you don't call."

(3) *Don't be accusatory.* "You care more about your work than about me!" is less effective than "I feel you're working too hard. Let's cut out of work early and hit a movie."

(4) *Tell her your perceptions.* "I feel I'm the only one who seems to initiate sex" is far less threatening than "You never try to seduce me anymore. You don't seem interested in sex!" (These communication skills are especially important when you're talking about sex.)

(5) *Don't interrupt each other.* It's one of the hallmarks of marital conversation that sends guys into a near-catatonic state. It'll drive her nuts too.

(6) *Tell her when you need space.* One buddy said, "After a hard day's work, I'd plop down in front of the TV. My wife would walk over, turn off the TV, and say, 'I find it offensive that you don't want to talk with me!' But it wasn't her. I was just too fried to talk to *anyone*, and I had to let her know I just needed time to chill. Once I spelled it out, she learned to wait for me to decompress."

Yeah, these basics are almost impossible to keep in mind all the time. But you will find yourself stopping your vicious attacks if you commit these points to memory.

146. You can finally stop dividing by two.

If you lived together, every time you had a fight, you started to divvy up possessions: "yours" and "hers." You can stop. In fact, if you don't stop, you'll remain separate—and marriage is nothing if not coming together, no holds barred. It's liberating; you sense the lines melting.

Count yourself blessed if your taste and your wife's are similar. You can buy together without freaking out. But the bigger part of making a home is what you edit. "I threw out half my stuff when I moved into her apartment," said my friend Sam. "But after we'd loaded up the station wagon five times, I looked at the remaining pile and said, 'I don't have the energy.'" Another friend called the process "healthy—but traumatic." A third had to do some serious negotiations for his prized collection of race car paintings. ("You can hang them in the bedroom," his new wife said, "but not the living room.") It gets picayune, down to the vitamins in the kitchen cupboard ("Out! And into the medicine cabinet!").

Don't be a control freak, like one guy who said to his new bride, "I don't want you bringing in a thing. Don't touch. Don't move. Don't alter." She said, "Can I breathe?" (She felt about as welcome as a cockroach; the marriage failed.) Be diplomatic. Another guy's attitude was, "You're living in my place. But it's our place. But it's still my place. All your furniture, it's junk— relatively speaking." She ended up in therapy and, amazingly, they worked past the problem together.

147. Plant some flags.

It's time for you two to mark your territory. If you were a team of explorers, the first thing you'd do when you reached new ground would be to stake your claim. You'd have a flag, an emblem, something that says, *We've Arrived! This is Ours! Pay Homage or Get Out!,* and you'd pound it mightily in the ground and toast your great, good fortune.

So, design your own logo. A sign for your house. Stationary with both your names. Come home with a slew of old photo frames, polish them with your wife, then stick You, the Couple photos in them and arrange them on a mantle, table, or piano. A shrine like this not only reminds you and your wife of your love, but sends a positive message to anyone who enters your home: *We're in love; treat us accordingly.*

Now create traditions. Invite family and friends for Thanksgiving, July 4th, or New Year's Day and make it H-O-M-E. My buddy Warren adopted his family's New Year's tradition of dressing in exotic costumes, then collecting paper scraps of everyone's worst and best memories of the previous year, plus their hopes and desires for the following year. He burned them in a cone as he marched around in the snow dressed as Father Time.

148. *Hide mementos from past girlfriends.*

This includes the wallet your French girlfriend gave you with the inscription "Je t'aime faire du fuck" on the inside; the framed photo of you smiling like a lunatic at the beach with an old girlfriend, both your necks covered with hickeys; the shoe box of college love letters in which a certain redhead promises to devour you; and the gift of boxer shorts with puckered red lips on the crotch.

Sometimes there's an item, a tie say, that could stay in your wardrobe. But you have the urge to confess that it was from a woman who you met on a train through Spain. Why would you want to tell her that? Because you hope to excite her jealousy, make her want you more, and get her looking over her shoulder (as if another woman is in line).

These and other bad dating habits can't be hauled onto marriage's decks—or they will sink the boat.

Don't feel guilty, however, when flickers of past girlfriends tickle your brain. The human mind is not like a garbage disposal: You can't flick a button and hear memories flush away.

149. Marriage will excite your bride's nesting instinct. And your hunter/gatherer instinct too.

While walking past a kitchen-supply store, my new wife pressed her head against the window and muttered, "It's beautiful." She was staring at a brushed aluminum four-burner gas stove—which startled me since she was using precisely the words and tone a guy uses when he spots the vintage Porsche of his dreams.

Frowning at the stoves, you feel yourself falling in line. Needless to say, you don't want to be like your predictable parents and the sleepwalkers who let marriage fly by.

While she's salivating over the appliances, you may find a new need to start whipping your yard into shape. I know I did. One night, I said to my wife, "Know what I'd really love? A lawn tractor." *A what?* "With an attachable wagon so I can haul a bush or tree around." *A what?* "So I can give our kids hay rides—someday." "Oh" she said.

I got my tractor. She got her stove.

MAKE YOUR BED THE EPICENTER OF YOUR NEW HOME. She needs an avalanche of pillows, so she feels feminine. You need something big, so you can pretend you're an Olympic gymnast scoring points by touching all four corners during a sex routine.

Splurge on new linens, pillows, and cases. If you come home

*one night with nifty new sheets, she will (guaranteed) call a girl-
friend to brag about your gift.*

---

150. Avoid home construction and major renovation when you're starting out in marriage.

It's rough enough to wage Construction War anytime. God forbid
you do it during your first year of marriage.

If normal marital arguments are playing with darts, then construction arguments are nuclear showdowns. Construction hits all
major marriage hot points: money, space, privacy, coordination,
gender roles, taste, decoration, authority. It turns you both into
ranting, raving lunatics.

In construction, nice guys finish last. You endure hardships—
then bite your spouse's head off. I've heard of workers who accidentally ripped a brand-new kitchen out of the wrong house and
tossed it in a dumpster. I've heard of workers snorting cocaine on
the bathroom tiles and then installing the ceramic soap dishes
upside down. I've heard of workers blow-torching the wrong pipes
together, so, after they leave, the water gushes out and destroys
months of labor.

You learn: Being a contractor means never having to say
you're sorry.

If you absolutely must do construction, hire a project manager (who will stand between you, the contractor, and his workers
like a hockey referee during a fight). Never go into a project without a complete contract (including a penalty fee schedule for late
work). Talk to your accountant or a financial planner in advance

to decide if you ought to refinance your mortgage or get a construction loan (which may be partially tax deductible).

One guy told me, "My wife and I have been through two renovations. And if you graphed our marriage the way they do the stock market, our renovations would look like Black Monday 1987 and the Tech Wreck 2000. Dismal."

151. Learn to compromise.

Once you're married, the microscope goes to high magnification. You have to learn the difference between each other's quirky habits and stuff that can be worked out through compromise. Here are two examples of quirky habits: She hates when you set your alarm so it will go off four times before you get up. Your justification: "So I can appreciate those last minutes of sleep." (This makes absolutely no sense to her.) You hate when she refuses to learn how to use more that two buttons on the TV remote control so she has to scroll through all fifty channels to return to the one you were watching previously. But you learn to laugh at those differences.

Compromise is different. And more complex.

Here's what many guys don't understand about compromise: It's not necessary to agree with everything your wife says or does. But you have to *think sincerely about why she feels the way she does.* Don't communicate like a guy I know, Mark: "Once my wife and I are talking about compromise, I really want to shut down. I don't believe in losing battles. Losing is a terrible thing. I feel like crashing through the door, leaving." Get it through your head: Compromise is not about losing.

Another guy recounted that he actually fell asleep while his wife was describing how to compromise on an issue (she threw socks at him, and he then denied he'd fallen asleep). OK, compromise is clearly tough for men. So how do you compromise?

Look for resolutions that make both partners feel they've gotten something important. For example, my friend Phil was obsessive about restoring or sailing his boat every day after work. His wife preferred lounging in one spot. She couldn't stand his scraping down the paint and laying down forty layers of varnish. ("The hull doesn't have to be like glass!!" she'd say.) So they compromised. He learned to sail shorter runs to nice beaches, where they'd both chill out. By the time they got back on the boat, she was ready to sail again.

152. Get organized.

To stay with the sailing metaphor, if you've ever sailed, you know the importance of having everything in order, so when there's a sudden wind shift, you're not fumbling to untie a tangled sheet.

It's the same in marriage. You bring two different systems (or lack thereof) into your marriage, and now is the time to unite them. Get equipped. Buy a box of manila folders, hanging files, labels, and either a file cabinet or accordion files. Get some easy-to-assemble cardboard file boxes so you can stash outdated, but-not-ready-to-throw-out papers in storage. Now get your system pat: one slot for your passports, one for your wills and estate planning, one for your lease or mortgage records, one for insurance forms, and on and on.

Next, think ahead to taxes. Get another file for receipts and organize them by category: utilities, telephone, entertainment, office expenses, charity, and so forth. Work together to keep your file up to date so there's no last-minute hysteria (which results in finger-pointing, accusations, and flared tempers).

Don't expect to have expertise in every area. Instead, hire a good accountant, lawyer, and all the rest.

Now think vacation. Clip articles and place them in a destination file, so you can plan ahead.

When you're done, get out the blender and mix up some margaritas.

153. Make plans.

After putting her through your indecision, she may be delivering you a glance that you know means, *Don't you dare get future-freaky on me again.*

The way to appease her trepidation is to create future dates. You need to be lured through time or you free fall, drift. It's like pitons in climbing.

But maybe you always dreaded a season's subscription to the symphony. (I did.) You feel too strapped in. Don't push your panic button. Know that a pair of theater or concert tickets wedged into her dressing mirror goes a long way toward showing that you're a committed guy. Stash air tickets for future vacations in her underwear drawer. Women need daily reminders that you're in it for the long run.

DON'T LOOK LIKE A TOTAL SLOB. Sometimes you go through an entire weekend in your rattiest clothes (or even worse, only under-

wear with worn elastic and inside-out, mismatched socks). You look at yourself in the mirror on Sunday night and realize that if you were a woman, you'd run the other way.

You knocked yourself out to find the right woman; now, don't turn her off.

---

154. Don't become decision impaired.

Lots of single guys are terrified that marriage will turn them into an Incapable-of-Knowing-What-I-Want. We watch, mouths agape, as a husband can't decide what to order at a restaurant. As a kid, I watched my best friend's mother read the menu to her husband like he was a baby. "Barry," she said, "I think you might like the chicken without the sauce." "What do you think about the salmon?" he asked. "The salmon could be OK." "I'll have the salmon," he said. "I really think you'd be happier with the chicken," she said. "I'll change that to the chicken," he said to the waiter. I thought, *This is pathetic! Doesn't this guy know what he wants to eat?*

What the hell is going on here? It comes from something good: day reporting. Thank God, you can finally have someone untangle what the hell happened to you that day. You get home, crack open a beer, and moan about office politics, work projects, and the rest. You discover pretty quickly that your wife has it all figured out. She sees right through everything. She predicts people's intentions because she understands their motives. It's uncanny. You begin to trust her opinion more than your own. Female intuition, savvy. You start to lean and then you lean and lean until you become a little boy asking what to eat.

Instead, use her as your secret weapon (appreciate her insights), but don't lose your taste buds over it.

155. Don't clam up.

I heard the same complaints about communication over and over from married women. "I just never know what he's thinking," one woman said. Another woman said, "How can he be my best friend if he doesn't talk and he's not listening? How can he be my soul mate? My girlfriends don't mind me going into detail or listening to my heartache. He's not one to get into the nitty-gritty of problems." And I heard, "He uses too few words. When he comes home from work, I say, 'How's your day?' and he says, 'Fine.' I say, 'Fine? That's all? Anything more?' 'Fine, Diane. Fine.' It's hard on me." Another woman said, "I hate when he says, 'What do you want from me?' or 'What did I do?' Or, worse, he'll freeze."

So, how do you open up? Some men need an activity. I can attest that some of the best conversations my wife and I ever had were while we were playing a lazy game of catch or walking on a beach. But you may need to try a few simple exercises. When you walk into the room after work, imagine you've changed roles. See yourself through her eyes. She's not trying to pry you open like an oyster; she's hoping to engage you, discover your world. "I know this sounds crazy, but sometimes I feel like my wife is trying to invade me," one guy said. "I go into a room and she follows. It's almost like an attack. She wants to know what I'm thinking, but *I* don't even know what I'm thinking. I'm trying *not* to think after a day of thinking." If that's the case, just tell her, "I just need a moment to decompress. It's not that I don't want to talk to you. It's just that I can't talk *at all* now." Sometimes all you need is time.

Give her a kiss, tell her you understand she wants to know what's going on, and that you'll get to it in a bit.

156. Don't complain endlessly about your work.

"I'm sure there are members of chain gangs who complain less about their work," one friend said to her husband.

"Oh," he said. "Got it."

But are you trying to show her your love through your work? "That doesn't turn me on," my friend Marina said. "It's easy for a guy to say he's going to take care of you and make so much money. But that's only money and real estate—and it takes a toll on a marriage.

"What *does* turn a woman on is when a guy has a grand plan, a vision of their life together. A grand plan is about shared adventure. It's about a guy including his woman in his dream. It's about a man being fulfilled. That might mean we live in a trailer home for a year while we convert an old barn into our home so we can live near his family and one day have huge Sunday dinners at a big table. Rather than living moment to moment, a grand plan means you have a picture in your heads of where you're going."

Sit down with your wife and two pads of paper. Write down your biggest life problem (no time, no creativity, no independence, or whatever) and a five-year solution (shorter than that, and you won't get there). Get down to the nitty-gritty of where you hope to live, how you hope to live, if you want to have kids, and the rest. Compare your visions. It may mean that you decide to live on an island for two years before you have kids so you don't go through life not having done it.

157. Yes, you are allowed to disagree.

We all know the guy who became glued at the hip to a woman. It's scary. They laugh in unison; say yes or no to the same things; never disagree; walk arm in arm (or hand in hand) in and out of parties; stand together; have the same friends, ideas, likes, and dislikes. "What wine will *we* have, Sweetie?" becomes yet another point of unification.

Ugh! What are they trying to suppress?! (Invariably, these are the couples who kiss for an entire airplane flight—and break up a month later.) They're afraid one disagreement will be taking the finger out of the dike, and . . . anarchy!

158. Try not to panic if you sense a door shutting.

It's sci-fi-like. You're in a room that's called Marriage, feeling fine, even dandy, when, slowly, you sense a door has shut. You listen. No noise. But wait: hissing. Hot steam. You suddenly realize all escapes have been closed. You loosen your tie, unbutton your top button, and soon you're yanking off your shirt, scratching the walls, and yelling for help. "Won't somebody get me outta here! Hello! Anyone there?! I can't breathe!!"

Your wife will say, "You seem distant" or "Is there something wrong?" or "I feel like you're not happy—and that makes me unhappy" or "I always thought we'd feel like one. But I've never felt so alone in all my life."

Know that many marriages start out shaky and get successively better. Don't throw in the towel. Don't say, "All my indecision was real! You didn't listen! I was right! There were real problems, and you were just too damned misty eyed about marriage to see it! It's your mother's fault! She pressured you, and you pressured me!"

Rather, crack open a few doors. Maybe you've (unnecessarily) sequestered yourself from your friends. There's an alraming tendency for some guys to give up that slide-in-the-mud soccer game soon after the wedding bells ring. Awful idea. If you surrender all your hunter/gatherer instincts, you'll feel feminized—and stomp out the door in search of a woman who makes you feel like a Neanderthal.

DON'T WAIT (UNTIL A DIVORCE) TO GET IN TOP SHAPE. Don't laugh. There's a type of guy who balloons up in marriage and seems to get divorced just so he can shed twenty-five pounds. (Each time he gets divorced, he stops eating steak, drinking scotch, and popping peanuts and potato chips into his mouth as if someone said they'd enhance sexual performance.) Then he drinks gallons of water each day, hits the gym, dumps his wardrobe, slides onto the dance floor, and meets the next wife—who will watch him blimp up again.

Instead, try the following prescription: Buy a pair of tight-fitting pants. Swear on the Bible you'll fit into these pants until you're six feet under. Throw them on at least once every twenty-one days. East and exercise accordingly.

159. *Define success on your own terms.*

It's a bit dicier to keep your perspective when guys barely past puberty are building twenty-five-thousand-square-foot houses with brick pizza ovens and a fourteen-burner stove.

I'm not worried about them; I'm worried about the rest of us. Married buddies told me, "I feel like I can't achieve anything in today's world." And: "All you hear about is the guy who just made a hundred million. I feel like I can't express my achievement. I can't keep up." One shrink said, "It's become a plague with men these days. All they think of is what they don't have—what the other guy has. Eight years ago, I never heard this in thcrapy, and now it's the first thing any man says. It's very disconcerting. It's almost like our society castrates men."

And it's not just money. Advertising seems to be out to get us—men—with all those pics of men with abs and pecs.

But for *your marriage* to be enough, you have to feel *you're* enough. Discuss all this with your wife. My wife constantly reminds me, "Money isn't everything." Or, when I become depressed over having missed the Next Big Opportunity, she says, "But that's not what we're after." All of which reminds me that I, too, sometimes fall prey to What Everybody Else Thinks *Is* Important.

Admittedly, it's a morose exercise, but imagine you were to die in a year. What would you want to do? Maybe you'd change careers or move out of the city or go to Opening Day at the ball park. One friend who actually had only a year to live told me, "All I ever wanted was to raise chickens." But he'd spent his life making millions in what he now saw as a meaningless activity. Understand what drives your wagon.

Now define success in marriage. One friend said he was walking down the street with his wife when she said, "You know, you're my best friend." And the next morning, he said to her, "I'm just glad to wake up next to you. You're my best friend, too." Success in marriage may be that simple.

160. *Close your eyes and fantasize about your dream job.*

Soon after he got married, my friend Ricky went into a room, shut off the lights, lay down, and decided he wanted to become a fly-fishing instructor. "Until I got married, I listened to my dad's advice: *Don't make your fun your business.* But once I was married, I did the opposite: I made my avocation my vocation. It was a dream I'd had since I was ten."

Ask your wife to do the same. You can help her bring sweeping changes to her work life, too.

161. *Surprise her.*

Grab her hand while you're walking past a spa and bring her in for a facial you've set up in advance. Or tape a note on her mirror, then another inside the medicine cabinet, and a third in her date book for her to find in the morning. Or scrub her feet while you're in the bath, then oil them when she's out of the bath, then oil her ankles, calves, and thighs. Then (and this is key), snuggle but don't insist on having sex. (She'll remember it more—or, if she's in the mood, let her initiate.)

Now get prepared so you can buy spontaneous gifts. Scribble down her sizes (for dresses, shoes, shirts, panties, bras, etc.) in your date book. Write down the names of her favorite saleswomen and stores, so you can pop in for a gift when the mood strikes you without having to call your wife for details.

One friend said, "When we were courting, I was such a regular at Victoria's Secret they would call when a new item came in. After we got married, for some reason I stopped—until one day, my wife said, 'What happened to all those bras you used to buy me?'"

162. Get used to wearing a ring.

Like many men, I'd never worn a ring before. I sensed its presence when I clapped or when I washed my face. I frequently toyed with the ring; it felt alien to my finger. Sometimes I'd pull it off to stare at our declaration of love on the inside. *Forever.*

On a powdery white beach in Thailand during our honeymoon, I toyed with my ring one time too many. Glossy with suntan oil, my thumb's pressure forced the ring to catapult off my finger like a tiddledywink and disappear into the fine sand. I froze. One step, and the ring might not be found for a thousand years. I called to my wife. From her lounge chair, she immediately detected the agony on my face. Luckily, we had befriended two Parisian archeologists who were also sunning nearby. "Attention, s'il vous plait," they said with authority, warning off beach strollers who came too close. Putting their skills to use, they drew an elaborate grid and emptied sand from one square and then the next. Villagers watched our obsessive efforts; a coconut vendor set up shop nearby. Two hours later, we uncovered the ring. Smiling Thai kids clapped as my wife placed the ring back on my finger; then we kissed with a curious mix of theatrical self-consciousness and sincerity: a wedding kiss.

After our honeymoon, I returned to the jewelry store. The

salesman agreed the ring was sized too big. We scaled it back without cutting into *Forever*. This time, my ring fit perfectly.

But the ring refused to stay on my finger where it belonged. Once, while blading through Central Park, a bee stung me literally underneath my wedding band. I had to have my ring sawed off after my finger ballooned to sausage proportions. Another time, while I was shoveling the front walk, my ring flew off my finger and landed somewhere in a foot of fresh snow. Despite hours sifting snow through a kitchen sieve, I couldn't find it (we searched into the night with a flashlight). The next morning, I took one step outside and there, frozen in the brittle ground, was the gleam of gold.

Eventually, you become *too* comfortable with your ring, and it slips into the landscape of your hand. Enliven it. Consider reenacting the ring ceremony on an anniversary. Exchange rings again. Renew vows.

We did just that on our tenth anniversary, dressed in T-shirts and sarongs (in honor of our Indonesian honeymoon) on a ridge overlooking our house, in a huddle with our two kids (and their two guinea pigs, Daniel and Paints). Was it the same as the first time? No. But marriage is about change. Overcome your fear that change in a relationship is bad.

BE CAREFUL OF THE MARRIED MAN REFLEX. That's when you're one hundred percent sure there's a single guy somewhere, some way, having a better time than you.

Getting wild with the woman you love is the best cure.

---

163. You will fight about the dumbest things—and that's part of marriage.

Like every couple, my wife and I have engaged in more idiotic fights than any statistician could count. But one fight stands out way above the rest for its sheer stupidity. We were en route to a much-anticipated, long-sold-out, Bob Dylan/Joni Mitchell concert when I said that Dylan was really in a different league from Mitchell—his songwriting genius was superior to her predictable, melodic repetition. My wife disagreed vehemently; suddenly, we were actually yelling, and before long, we were really discussing the merit of Penis Music versus Vagina Music.

What made it doubly irritating was that Dylan (notorious for his erratic performances) was awful and Mitchell was brilliant. Score: Vaginas 1, Penises 0. I kept rooting for him to wake up, but he seemed only to get more nasal. "Unless Joni's coming back out to rescue him, let's go," my wife said. I agreed. Vaginas 2, Penises 0.

It's not the fights that count; it's the recoveries. There's a point where you have to come back together and laugh at yourself.

Besides, it's not the couples who argue who are in trouble; it's those who don't who hit the skids.

164. Stay alert for repeats in your fighting repertoire.

Too many fights have a familiarity to them. She asks you to pick up groceries on your way back from the gym, and you always forget—which sends her a message that you find vanity more important than domesticity. "We're not fighting about what's really wrong," one friend said. "It's usually that we haven't spent enough time together or we're frustrated about other things."

When you can practically recite the lines to your fight before you have it, it's time to get your act together.

165. Know when to stop knocking yourself out to please your mother-in-law.

It's important not to bend too far backward for certain mothers-in-laws, or you may get a gentle nudge.

My friend Rick said that early in his marriage he tried almost too hard to please his mother-in-law. "Boxwoods are my mother-in-law's favorite shrub," he told me. "So, I thought I'd win major points for planting them as a hedge. Knowing of our friction, my wife called her mother and said, 'Rick planted a bunch of boxwoods out front.' Suddenly, I was being handed the phone. My mother-in-law said, 'Are they American boxwood?' 'Ah . . . no. Actually, they're Korean boxwood,' I said. Silence. Then: 'Can I speak with my daughter?' It was as if I'd said I was having an affair with a Korean woman! And then I was having it out with my wife because her mother is impossible to please!"

Remember, what's at stake here is Who Treats Her Daughter Better: Mommy or You. Try not to place your wife in the middle. It's best if you can joke about it. Then, stand your ground with your mother-in-law.

166. End arguments with sex.

Sex is more than a Band-Aid. If your marriage is a record and a fight is hitting the same groove over and again, then sex can be the gentle nudge that gets you unstuck. You discover once again what brought you together in the first place, then you attack the problem together—not from opposite sides. One female friend said, "When things get really stressful, I look at my husband and say, 'Honey, let's go fuck.' He will get the biggest smile on his face—and later we hash out the details of our disagreement."

167. Never shoot your mouth off thoughtlessly.

"I'd rather discover that you're having an affair than find a $2,500 charge on your Bloomingdale's card," said my friend Vanessa's husband to her between bites of tortilla chips and salsa. My wife and I looked aghast—but Vanessa looked devastated. She went white, then red. "You mean," she said, setting down her sangria, "my fidelity is only worth twenty-five hundred bucks to you?" He protested, "Hon, don't get me wrong." She replied in a high-pitched voice: "But that's how you feel?"

"Yeah, it's how I feel. It takes a hell of an effort to earn twenty-five hundred bucks. And I know our marriage could survive an affair. It's meant as a compliment."

Well, it wasn't taken as a compliment. (Everyone at the table thought, *He must have had an affair, or he'd never say such a thing.*)

Don't say anything even half as dumb.

168. Don't turn her positives into negatives.

My friend Piet said, "When we were dating, one of the things I liked most about my now-wife was her inability to tolerate small talk. She would rather prune a rose bush than engage in idle chitchat. But when we were married, I found myself criticizing the very quality I most adored. 'You hate to socialize!' I yelled one night. 'Don't you ever need to go to parties?!' She turned to me and said, 'Who'd you think you were marrying? A sorority girl?'

"And she was right. I'd known other women who liked to socialize. Then I began to enjoy my wife's ability to entertain herself again. It's calming."

169. Be lovers.

Not to denigrate companionship, but what we all hunger for is to remain lovers.

Physical intimacy is more than frosting on the cake; it is the cake. What distinguishes your marriage from all your other friendships and family relationships is physical intimacy. Give up being lovers, and you've joined the ranks of other endangered married couples.

Now understand some of the differences between men and women when it comes to sex. Men need sex to feel good about ourselves. Women need to feel good about themselves before sex. Men need sex to relax. Women need to be relaxed to enjoy sex. Men are visual when it comes to sex. With women, it's intimacy.

(Aside from that, we're exactly the same.)

170. Everybody makes too much of making the bed, setting down the toilet seat, and neatly folding the toothpaste tube.

You can try to be the Rebel of Toilet Seat Etiquette, but it's not going to win you many female hearts. My friend Howard said, "Why aren't guys allowed to be equally irritated that women are constantly leaving the toilet seat down? Why do I always have to move it up, then back down? Why is it a woman's right to find the seat down every time?"

Try falling into a toilet bowl in the middle of the night, and you'll know why.

Don't laugh at this little stuff (it's more tied to your sex life than hormones). "It turns me off when my husband leaves his towels all crumpled up on the floor. I feel like the motel maid!" one female friend said. "He just doesn't get it!" But nobody has bothered to tell guys that the two most important qualities for a man in marriage are (1) his ability to clean a kitchen and (2) his ability to clean a bathroom.

171. If oral sex is your thing, don't stop in marriage.

You hear the same male complaint over and over: "She was so into oral sex. Then I proposed. Then we got married. Then it was over." Are all men genetically programmed to complain about the lack of oral sex? Or are we expecting too much?

But before we figure out the solution, let's ask why oral sex is so important to guys? The answer: We like to watch. Men are visual creatures. We enjoy pleasure, but we enjoy the *sight* of pleasure even more. And the sight of oral sex is for a man what a luminous sunset is to the folks at Hallmark cards.

We're also turned on by the idea that only we know how much of a wild woman our wife can be. "When I was a kid," one friend said, "nothing I fantasized about ever seemed to come true. *Playboy* Bunnies didn't leap off the pages and onto my lap. Beautiful women shunned me at every turn. One of the things I like about marriage is that my fantasies with my wife *can* come true. When I'm at a staid business party, I know what we can do later that night, and it makes the tedium of nodding and smiling at everyone almost tenable."

So how do you keep oral sex in your marriage? Several important rules, culled from my friends who've managed to keep that particular zip in their marriages: (1) giveth unto her if thou would like to receiveth (and listen to her instructions, so you know her terrain); (2) take a shower beforehand; (3) stop holding her head (unless she's a porno queen, she probably doesn't appreciate the gesture, and if she is a porno queen, you're probably not married to her).

172. *Really kiss your wife.*

I was standing in a quarter inch of beer at Madison Square Garden to hear a Jimmy Page-Robert Plant concert when I noticed a young couple a row in front moving into explore-the-cosmos kisses (heads twisting, tongues down each other's throats) with each song. Married couples kiss like this when they're making love (sometimes), but almost never when they're not having sex, and *never* in public.

When was the last time you two stopped at a street corner and kissed?

173. *Tell her with your eyes.*

Remember how in courtship you used to stare into each other's eyes, and then she'd say, "I know," or "I feel the same way?" All that abruptly ends in marriage—and it shouldn't.

And then there's eye contact while making love. When you're facing her, open your eyes, comb her hair, don't say a word.

•   •   •

174. Redefine the quickie.

Not every time you have sex will be like a Mark McGuire home run: a towering shot to center, dropped jaws, time stops.

As long as it's mutually understood, you have to bring a new tune into your repertoire: the quickie. Example: you've got fifteen minutes until your guests arrive for dinner, and you're both still naked in the bathroom; go for it (you greet the guests while she puts on her makeup). My friend Bev said, "Fifteen minutes!? How about two?! We giggle and laugh about it. We'll do it on the bathroom floor with guests downstairs having a glass of wine!"

175. Don't masturbate so much you have no appetite for sex with your wife.

One married friend said, "I beat off so much in the shower I can barely walk to breakfast." OK, he's got kids (and kids to morning sex are what a hail storm is to a tennis match). And granted, every guy can double click and be over the porno rainbow. And stress seems to be the glue that holds our world together. And we need a temporary reprieve.

But it's vital that you stay hungry for her. Sometimes that means telling Rosy Palm to take the day off.

176. Make sex a priority.

I'm not saying you ought to postpone bill paying until the creditors are knocking on your door, but sometimes, the bills will have to wait because sex is more important. More important than raking the leaves, putting up the storm windows, or cleaning out your storage attic.

Soon into marriage, you realize that exhaustion is the enemy.

Stress is the enemy. "No time!" is the enemy. Which means, hit the hay early, clean the slates, erase the day, create time. Sooner or later (and probably sooner), she'll resent sex if you start at 11:30 P.M. or midnight. "Sometimes, I feel like I've been asked to do too many things all day, and I can't do one more thing," my friend Julia said. "At eleven o'clock, I just need to go to sleep."

Almost all the couples I spoke with who profess to have good sex lives have one thing in common: They allow themselves to be seduced, even when they're not in the mood at first. They're also good at giving each other time to decompress. One woman said, "I feel like I wear a jock strap all day at work, and then have to switch into lingerie at home. With all the pressures, it's not an immediate transition."

FIND HER FAVORITE TIME TO MAKE LOVE. (It may not be nighttime.) Then: adapt!

---

177. Stop reading sex surveys.

Magazine covers boast, "New Findings!" and ask, *Are you good enough? Is it frequent enough? Does it last long enough? Are her orgasms good enough? Powerful enough? Are her orgasms vaginal or clitoral? (Or both at once?!) And what about multiple orgasms!? And are you having multiple orgasms?* Read up and worry: *Some men have multiple orgasms every time!* Or, the contradictory article: *Male orgasms bring on premature aging. After age thirty-five, one orgasm per sixty days is about right.* (That number may have been OK for ancient monks, but with today's stress, wouldn't we explode?)

And if you really want to worry, start reading how you should alter your diet so your semen tastes . . . yum! (No garlic, tomato, or coffee.)

The world wants you to turn sex into a comparison sport. Don't go there.

DON'T OBSESS OVER FREQUENCY. One guy actually bought a pin cushion and stuck in a pin each time he and his wife had sex during Year One. During Year Two, he pulled out a pin after they had sex. "We'd better get rolling," he said, when he realized there were too many pins still in the cushion.

His wife thought he was nuts.

---

178. Be vocal.
A married woman adores it when you still say you love her *while* having sex.

179. Don't be threatened by her fantasies—or make her pay for them afterward.
Contrary to popular rumor, women have wonderfully dirty minds.

Ask her, and if she feels safe from retribution, she'll tell you. Stable fantasies. Horse fantasies (on a horse, by a horse, with you looking; on a horse, by a cowboy wearing nothing but chaps, with you masturbating). Pizza-delivery-boy fantasies (he brings everything but the pizza). Shy man-with-glorious-penis fantasies.

The problem is morality. You hear these fantasies and get off on them (wildly), then you get crazed with propriety. *What sort of woman did you marry?* You feel inadequate (unless you're a horse or a cowboy in nothing but chaps).

But if you let her whisper those fantasies to you, she'll trust you more, your sex will be vivid, and you'll be part of that elite group of men: the liberateds. Her fantasies would have been inappropriate while you were getting to know her, but now that you're married, there's a chance to go further. Buy her sexy lingerie, so she can feel like a prettily decorated gift. ("I go by that old dictum," one female friend said, "I wanna be a lady on the street and a whore in bed.") You can even hitch her fantasies to one of your own: watch her masturbate. You can practically hear her mind purr.

Go for it.

WRITE "I LOVE YOU" ON HER PAPER COFFEE CUP WHEN YOU COME BACK FROM THE DELI. Your wife will adore it when you proclaim your love in casual—and unexpected—ways.

---

180. Stop getting ready for sex.

You take off your clothes. She takes off hers. You hang them or fold them or toss them in the hamper. She wraps herself in a towel. You slip under the covers. Wow! It's—all—so—dull.

Regularity sucks. Take a glance back at those heady days when she used to gyrate against your jeans leg, and you used to yank off her sweater and T-shirt and unbutton her pants. Do whatever it takes. Turn your order upside down.

181. Temptation happens.

To keep sane, learn the following rules:

1. *Know when to slam on the brakes.* My friend Eric, now married, was on a business trip, alone and luxuriating in a rooftop Jacuzzi, staring at the full moon, when a woman shed her robe and got in with him. It turned out that she was a struggling actress, and she leaned her head back, as if to say, *Go ahead. Admire the water gurgling over my breasts.* She got out, dried herself off, and asked him to walk her back to her room. "I walked her back," Eric said. "Then she invited me in. An alarm went off. I thought, *This will be a chink in the china you'll never fix.* I took a deep breath and said, 'Goodnight.' "

2. *Create little moments of discovery.* Another friend said, "Not immediately, but soon after I was married, my head really started turning. I wanted what I couldn't have. When I'd walk to work, I'd spot a dozen women and wonder what it would be like to see them peel off their clothes for me. But when I stopped to think about it, it wasn't really about sex. I realized I missed the little moments of discovery that we had early in our relationship. For instance, seeing her walk naked to fix the morning coffee. Or having her wear my shirt with nothing underneath." The solution is to keep those moments in your relationship—and it starts with you. Treat her like she's sexy.

3. *Don't get freaked out by statistics on adultery.* Aside from complexity (one guy said, "I'm constantly tripping over my lies"),

affairs undermine the integrity of your marriage. Your marriage can be whatever you want: a shack or a palace. But it can't be both.

4. *Ignore the rationalizations of men who have affairs.* You'll hear things like, "I go under the assumption that if a tree falls in a forest and nobody hears, it didn't happen." And "You only go around the track once, and I don't want to have regrets." And "I have no problem with commitment. I'm committed to many, many women." When I told one guy what these men had said, he retorted, "Yeah, they say that stuff so they can sleep well at night."

5. *Forget about the arguments of men who try to challenge your monogamy.* During my first year of marriage, an old high school buddy, who'd been married since his early twenties, took me out for a beer and "confessed" that he has thirty affairs per year. "I'm not sure if I've slept with four digits," he murmured. "Four digits?" I asked. "Over a thousand women," he said, smiling and leaning back in his chair. "You have three kids," I said. He nodded. "And a nine-to-seven job," I said. He nodded. "So, when do you have the time?" I asked. He looked at the ceiling and replied, "I *make* the time." All this tested my mathematical abilities. I calculated his age, minus his age when he presumably lost his virginity, multiplied by 365 (days per year), and then divided by his number of screwings to arrive at his daily average. (Later that night, I told my wife about my high school chum's bed habits, and she said, "Yuck! Who would want to sleep with a thousand of anything?")

6. *Realize that most of the single guy chest-pounding isn't as grand as it first seems.* Once, on the ski lift for my first run of the

day, I asked the guy beside me, "So, how's the snow?" "Well, I guess I didn't notice," he said, yawning. "See, I spotted a beautiful woman at a restaurant last night, asked her to join me for a glass of wine, took her back to my condo, and didn't sleep hardly a wink the entire night. The chick loves sex. So, I catch an hour of shut-eye, then she wakes me up by giving me a blow job. I can barely walk, man. That woman nearly screwed me to death."

For a moment, I felt as all married men do: a brief flicker of envy.

But I learned as we rode farther up the lift that he'd left his wife and kid. ("It rips my heart out to call my son," he said. "He can't stand my guts.") "You've got it made," he told me as we got off the lift.

He was right.

NO, YOU CANNOT ASK YOUR WIFE, "CAN I HAVE A SECOND WIFE— JUST FOR SEX?" It's astonshing how many women reported to me that their husbands asked that very question. Some women replied, "Come again?!" Others wanted details: "Will she cook and clean? Will she do the laundry? Can she go clothes shopping for me? Can she stand around and look good so I can chew gum and wear sweat pants all the time?"

I asked the obvious follow-up question: "Wouldn't you want a second husband—just for sex?" "No," they all agreed. "That would be too much male energy in the house."

Hmmm . . .

182. Flirt if you must.

That poor, ol' underutilized reptilian part of your brain wants to know you could still attract a chick if you had to. It's like practicing archery, so you know you could hunt for deer if urban civilization crumbled.

You spot a beautiful woman at a bookstore. You track her while she moves to a display table. Now she pretends she hasn't spotted you. She flicks her hair *(attraction),* smiles and then lifts a book *(come get me).* You move beside her and lift another copy of the same book, and she turns ever so slightly toward you *(I'm all yours).* You open with something plausible ("You read any reviews on this book?")—she has—and suddenly, you're off to the races with loaded, frothy, excited, bubbly talk. It's almost as if you have flicked a switch in your brain. *If there weren't such a thing as commitment and marriage had never been invented and "other women" meant "pastrami" and "adultery" meant "rye" and "infidelity" meant "mustard", I'd sit down to have my favorite sandwich.* Then she looks toward the door *(beam me home, Scotty).*

But talk is cheap and a cappuccino's right over there—and after five minutes, you've proved you can still hunt. OK, Cave Boy, time to get back to the cave and funnel all that sexual energy toward the woman you love.

NO, AN INTERNET AFFAIR IS NOT A HARMLESS FLIRTATION. Don't fool yourself. If you're slobbering over your keyboard while you're pecking sultry salutations to a babe in Boise, you're betraying the trust of the woman you love.

Guys tend to define an affair as Penis Enters Vagina. Uh-uh. Need proof? One woman told me that nearly the instant her husband got married, he began sending hot-and-bothered Internet notes to a woman in cyberspace. He then told his wife he was going on a business trip. He went instead to visit the woman behind the moaning computer notes. He moved out from the wife and in with the Internet lover. (Naturally, he cheated via Internet on her, too.)

OK, the guy's a psycho. But it's called Distancing. Don't distance yourself from the woman you love.

---

183. Now flirt with your wife.

Marital talk can get so dull. Yes means yes and no means no and maybe means, "I can't be bothered." It's just one hell of a lot harder to flirt when you've seen each other up, down, and all around for years.

My friend Frank says, "I tell my wife to get dressed up with nothing on underneath. Then we meet like two strangers for dinner. I walk into the restaurant, and there she is sitting at the bar. She's beautiful. Other men are eyeing her from across the room. I'm totally turned on."

WHEN THE GOING GETS TOUGH, THE TOUGH GO TO A HOTEL. *A night away is cheaper than an hour of couple's therapy—and a hell of a lot more fun. Or take an hour off work to meet her. Married men do this stuff with their mistresses every day—so why not do it with your wife?*

184. Have an affair—with your wife.

Here's a rule of marriage you can't know too soon: Your marriage will need the zippity-zap, electric jolt of an affair. But you're going to be creative. You're going to take the time and energy to have knockout, upside-down, head-turning affairs with your wife.

One friend, who'd been married about a year, recounted how they were ready to snap each other's heads off before they went to a hotel for a night. "We'd been under a lot of stress. That morning, we fought, and she called me at work to say we ought to cancel. But we went through with it. I had no expectations whatsoever.

"Then everything changed just picking her up in the car. My wife had worn her leather pants and a tight new shirt. The instant we closed the hotel room door, we poured wine into each other's mouths and then we were all over each other. It felt new and nasty. Neither of us could believe how hot it was. The sex put that great glow over everything; at dinner, she ran her hand under the table and up my leg for the first time in years. The next day, I had to be back at work by noon—but I felt we'd been away for weeks."

It's especially important to go away with your wife when your marriage seems tired. Bring a few bottles of her favorite wine, incense, candles, the right music, and bath oil or body lotion. You know the stuff. Don't forget the down-and-dirty props if that's your thing (magazines, video, toys). If you don't rip each other's clothes off once you're in the room, start with a back rub. And don't open up mail, read the paper, or watch the news. (One buddy reported bringing along a letter, which turned out to be an IRS audit notification. "My wife lay in the bath while I consulted with my accountant. It was a total waste of time and money. We went home angry and anxious.")

Here's when you'll *really* need these affairs: (1) when adversity strikes and (2) when you have kids. I know a couple who went through a tough time. The husband said, "We'd never have made it if not for little pockets of time where we reminded ourselves of why we loved each other. Four or five hotel nights in a year saved our marriage."

Set up good marriage patterns now. It's akin to spinning your legs on a bike *before* you hit the steep incline: forward motion propels you.

YOUR LOVE WILL GO IN AND OUT OF FOCUS. You will go into periods where your wife seems distant and vague. And then, all of a sudden, you will look at her and see, with blinding clarity, the woman you fell in love with. To me, this is the payoff nobody seems to mention when they talk about love. It's falling in love all over again, and again, that makes marriage work.

---

185. Create sacred spaces.
Your bedroom ought to be one. Invent more.

One place my wife and I revere is our vegetable patch. It's amazing in fall, when the tomatoes are dwindling and we stand among two dozen pumpkins. With leaves twirling through the air, we get the rush of head-over-heels love again.

Or you may have a sacred song. My friend Dan promised his wife that every time they heard the sound track from *Ghost*, he would stop whatever he was doing and dance with her. ("It's one thing when we're in the kitchen, but another when he pulls off when we're driving and dances with me on the side of the road," she said.)

That's the stuff that keeps a marriage going.

186. For your marriage to work, you'll need an hour, plus an hour, per day.

The first hour is solo time—for you. (Aside from work or bill paying.) Just one hour to find yourself, get your center, chill. (No, you don't have to be staring at the ceiling; exercising, walking, playing music, or reading will do the trick.)

The second hour is together time—with your wife. Once again, logistical stuff doesn't count. Think along the lines of talking, cooking, laying under a tree, or taking a bath.

You think a marriage can survive without daily down time (alone and together)? Think again. You're not being selfish if you need time to be alone. Men need to swing out into the world to whirl back in. It's our nature; don't go against it. And women need time alone, too.

187. Be hopelessly romantic.

Early in their marriage, my friend Bev's husband borrowed his wife's address book, and returned it with a love note written atop each page: "A, because you're awesome. B, because you're beautiful. C, because you're clever. D, because you're delectable. E, because you're everything to me. F, because you fulfill my needs. G, because you're great in the sack. H, because I can't get you out of my head . . ."

"My address book is my favorite possession in the whole world," Bev said. "I'll read it to Dan when we're having troubles (he jokes that he never wrote it). It keeps us on course."

188. Don't believe in the concept of an ideal mate.

It's yet another Hollywood-induced illusion. What is an ideal mate? Is anyone ideal? You and your wife may have a terrific marriage, but if it's not ideal, what are you to do? Dump her for a younger chick who might be ideal?

**Trash all the glossy lingo and you'll have a better chance of enjoying your marriage.

189. Forget fairy-tale endings.

"I always thought, *Once I've got my man, it'll be great,*" my friend Dana said. "I'll be a lovable person. But a few months into marriage, I thought, *This is it? This was going to save me? This was going to make it all OK?*"

There is no such thing as "And they lived happily ever after." Neither of you can wake up each day dreaming that you've married the person who will erase sadness from your life. But both of you *have* married the person who will stick with you through thick and thin. If you move past the neat ending, you become partners. You thrive on your own *and* with each other.

•   •   •

190. *Realize that the day will come when you cannot imagine not being married.*

It was a glistening fall day, and a good friend was getting married on a bluff over the Hudson River. A sea of white roses. Pleasant anticipation. And (typically): a delay.

I kissed my wife and then strolled to the other side of a gazebo, where the groom was pacing. "What's the story, bucko?" the groom said with a nervous smile. "Am I making the mistake of a lifetime? Is this marriage thing OK—for a guy?"

I glanced over at my wife and remembered my years of indecision. All of it—the fears, fights, and toil—seemed distant, even ridiculous. Sure, our marriage had its bumps, like any marriage. But I realized I wouldn't trade it for what I had then. "No, man," I said, "you're doing the right thing." The music began. He gave me a last bear hug, and I dashed to my seat beside my wife.

As we watched them walk the aisle, my wife and I felt nostalgic (as all couples do when they realize they're no longer newlyweds). We held hands. Quietly, I slipped her ring off her finger. She looked at me, slightly aghast. When I slipped it back on, she kissed me softly and lay her head on my shoulder.

And I whispered, "Forever . . ."

Acknowledgments

THANKS TO Henry Ferris, my editor; Elizabeth Kaplan, my agent; and everyone at HarperCollins, including Susan Weinberg, Michael Morrison, Lisa Queen, and Jennifer Hart. I am grateful to Elizabeth Pawlson, Leslie Cohen, and Sharyn Rosenblum for their tireless work on my behalf.

Special thanks to Miriam Cohen. I have benefited greatly from her encouragement and wisdom.

I appreciate Deborah Matlovsky's advice and insight. Andrew Lund made a great contribution with his Guy Think and intelligence.

I received invaluable female feedback from Ruti Artis, Allison Berglas, Adrienne Farb, Gayle Grabell, Elin McCoy, Abigail Ross, and Patty White. I am grateful to John Frederick Walker for his critical readings. Thanks to my parents, Lynn and Steve, for the gift of their forty-seven-year (and going strong) marriage. Warm thanks to the many interviewees for their vivid commitment stories.

But the grand-finale fireworks, jets flying in formation, Eiffel Tower at sunset, and flowing champagne go to my wife and kids. To Jeannette, for knowing all along that we should spend our life together; to Isabelle for saying, "Your wedding looks like so much fun! Why couldn't I have been there?" and to Benjamin for saying, "I might read this book before I get married."